GROW
HAIR
FAST

7 Steps to a New
Head of Hair in 90 Days

Riquette Hofstein

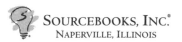

SOURCEBOOKS, INC.®
NAPERVILLE, ILLINOIS

Copyright © 2004 by Riquette Hofstein
Cover and internal design © 2004 by Sourcebooks, Inc.
Sourcebooks and the colophon are registered trademarks of Sourcebooks, Inc.

All rights reserved. No part of this book may be reproduced in any form or by any electronic or mechanical means including information storage and retrieval systems—except in the case of brief quotations embodied in critical articles or reviews—without permission in writing from its publisher, Sourcebooks, Inc.

This book is not intended as a substitute for medical advice from a qualified physician. The intent of this book is to provide accurate general information in regard to the subject matter covered. If medical advice or other expert help is needed, the services of an appropriate medical professional should be sought.

Published by Sourcebooks, Inc.
P.O. Box 4410, Naperville, Illinois 60567-4410
(630) 961-3900
FAX: (630) 961-2168
www.sourcebooks.com

Library of Congress Cataloging-in-Publication Data

Hofstein, Riquette.
  Grow hair fast / by Riquette Hofstein.
      p. cm.
  Includes index.
  ISBN 1-4022-0257-1 (alk. paper)
  1. Hair—Growth. 2. Hair—Care and hygiene. I. Title.
RL91.H668 2004
                                                    646.7'24—dc22

Printed and bound in the United States of America
VP 10 9 8 7

To my parents, Jacques and Sarah Hofstein, on
their 60th wedding anniversary. For their total love and
understanding, and for allowing me to grow and discover who
I really am, without question and with total trust.

Author's Note

All plants, like all medicines, may be dangerous if used improperly. If they are taken internally when prescribed for external use, or if they are taken in excess or over too long a time, allergic reactions and unpredictable sensitivities may develop.

To determine whether you are allergic to any of the recipes in this book, test preparations on a small patch of skin before using them on the hair, scalp, or face.

Every effort has been made to ensure that the recipes and substances used in this book are safe when used as directed.

Keep herbs fresh and conditions of use as sterile as possible.

Acknowledgments

First and foremost, I would like to thank all of my clients who are the daily fulfillment of my life's purpose. I would also like to thank the individuals who assisted so wholeheartedly with this book—Jan Nathan of Publishers Marketing Association, who introduced me to my publishing house; Deb Werksman, my editor at Sourcebooks; Gerry Bryant for his excellent advice. And I am eternally thankful for the everlasting knowledge of my professors who have supported and inspired me since my days studying health and nutrition. May all your dreams transpire, your hearts embrace, and your hair grow.

Table of Contents

Introduction

My goals for this book are threefold: to educate, motivate, and stimulate your mind on a subject I am fiercely passionate about—hair care. I fully realize that a book is merely a tool, but books have been known to make big changes in the people who read them. I would like you to think of this book as an experience that could very well change your life.

I have been licensed in the field of trichology (the study of hair and roots) for over thirty years. I opened my first clinic in 1969 in Sydney, Australia, and eventually started my company, *Riquette International,* after moving to Beverly Hills in 1981. I have seen and helped thousands of clients who come to me from all walks of life. Some of them are movie stars, rock stars, politicians, and executives in Fortune 500 corporations, while others range across the socioeconomic spectrum to children and single mothers working at the convenience store around the corner. Many of them walk through my door as a last-ditch effort, acting out of fear and desperation over the loss of, or severe damage to, their hair. Their stories are often sad and poignant cases, replete with shame, anger, and shattered self-esteem.

The information presented within these pages is derived from the very same techniques and methods I have employed to successfully (some would say miraculously) turn the proverbial ship around for my clients. The results have been astonishing. I have files and files of heartfelt letters of gratitude from my clients, thanking me for accomplishing what they all firmly believed was an absolute impossibility.

I really have a lot of compassion for the people who come through my doors. I completely identify with their deep-set anguish and injured dignity. *Really.*

I've been there. I know what it's like.

I was born in Cairo, Egypt, to my very sweet and dear parents, Jacques and Sarah Hofstein. By the time we moved to Paris when I was eight, I already knew what I wanted to do. There was a hairstyling academy not too far from our home. My parents, who were always encouraging my sister, Paulette, and me to try new things, easily agreed to allow me to go and hang around the academy. I met the headmaster and talked him into letting me run errands for the instructors. I have no idea what he thought of this precocious little girl who was so eager to work for no money, but he let me stay and listen to the lectures in exchange for the errands. And listen I did.

When my parents moved our family to Sydney, I immediately enrolled in a four-year apprenticeship at Alexander of Alexander International Hairdressers. I was fourteen and still in school. My parents were extremely supportive. Mummy would pick me up from school every day and cart me off to Alexander, then wait for me until I was finished. At night she would be my model, allowing me to cut, perm, color, and do just about anything you could imagine. Papa even got into the act by allowing me to practice scalp massages and rolling curlers in his wavy, silky black hair.

After receiving my BA from the Beauty Technical College in Sydney, I avidly continued my education by studying at the

Schwarzkopf Institute of Hair Research in Munich, London's Max Factor Makeup School, the International College of Aesthetics in Rome, Geneva's famous skin care institute La Prairie, and I earned my certification in trichology from the prestigious René Furterer Institute in Paris. Eventually I received advanced degrees and certifications in makeup, hair and skin care, hypnosis, nutrition, iridology, holistic healing, and stress management in over fourteen European countries and North America.

My studies were as much an academic endeavor as they were a personal journey for answers. During my teenage years I was afflicted with a terrible and emotionally debilitating case of acne. At times, it was so awful that I believed that all anyone could see on my face was my eyes. To make matters worse, my hair became so brittle and fragile that it began to fall out. My parents took me to a series of doctors, and I consulted every dermatologist I could find. No one had the answer to healing my condition.

Finally, I came to the realization that if anyone was going to figure this out, then it would probably have to be me. I had to learn to trust myself, and take all my advanced training to a heretofore-unexplored territory. I began experimenting with altering my diet, taking vitamin supplements, and using herbs. This was back in the days when the field of herbology was still very new and regarded with a great deal of skepticism. My travels throughout the world brought me in direct contact with a lot of stories and folklore about the use of herbs in curing the body of ailments. I tried them all—in every combination I could think of. Eventually, I did find the answer. My skin cleared up, and my hair became more lush, beautiful, and healthy than ever before.

Then I made an intuitive leap that changed my life: if it worked for me, surely it will work for someone else. A lucid understanding of the greater purpose and meaning for my life washed over me. I had found my passion: to educate, motivate, and stimulate other people toward their optimal beauty, vitality, and health. This book represents a major step toward the fulfillment of that life purpose.

1

First Impressions:

Hair's Intimate Connection to Our Personal Identities

In the summer of 1991, high in the Tyrolean Alps of Northern Italy, a team of archeologists and other scientists retrieved the preserved body of a man buried in the glacial fields. First impressions led the body's discoverers to assess that he was a hiker who had been caught in an avalanche and had perhaps only been dead for four or five decades at most. Upon closer inspection of his clothes and tools, the team adjusted the estimate of his date of death to almost fifty-three hundred years before!

What gave the impression that this Neolithic mummy, now known as the Iceman, had been an inhabitant of the twentieth century? In short, it was his *hair*—the manner in which it was cut and the fact that his beard was trimmed to boot.

The Iceman has revealed much about life at the dawn of the Copper Age, including the fact that our modern concern with appearances, particularly when it comes to hair, is not by any means a new sociological development. Indeed, a cursory examination of civilization throughout the ages will show that hair, how it appears and how styles have evolved, has always been an important part of our development as a species.

The way we wear our hair is closely tied to the times we live in and to the society into which we are born. As new hairstyles develop and emerge, you can be certain that substantial cultural changes are taking place.

Remember when Farah Fawcett rose to stardom with her feathered mane and virtually every woman in Western civilization raced to her hairdresser? What else was going on in society but the Sexual Revolution? Remember when Demi Moore emerged as a superstar in *Ghost*? After that movie's opening weekend, every woman in America started asking for the same cut Demi had. Women were just beginning to make their mark as independent spirits climbing the ladder of a booming corporate economy. And when Bruce Willis debuted with his buzz-cut opposite Cybill Shephard in *Moonlighting* while Don Johnson worked the streets with a stubble beard in *Miami Vice*, America turned toward massive consumerism and junk bonds during the Reagan Years. That was quickly followed by radical hairstyles from Cyndi Lauper, Madonna, and Flock of Seagulls as a sort of antiestablishment answer to what was going on in the mainstream.

Rock musicians and movie stars have not been the only purveyors of fashion when it comes to how we wear our hair. Politicians, aristocrats, and religious leaders throughout the centuries have had a profound influence on the culture of hair. From the Pharaohs of Egypt to the first Caesar of Rome to the monks of the Middle Ages to Louis the XIV (who adopted the fashion of wearing powdered wigs to cover his balding crown), hair has always been closely tied to the evolution of world society.

When Samson, a man of apparently insuperable strength and power, fell in love with the Philistine Delilah, we are told that his head was adorned with seven long braids—he had been forbidden by God to ever submit to a haircut. Delilah was charged by Samson's copious enemies with the duty of discerning the key to his downfall. After several failed attempts, she beguiled him into revealing his secret: "There hath not come a razor upon mine head," he said, "for I have been a Nazarite unto God from my mother's womb: if I be shaven, then my strength will go from me, and I shall become weak, and be like any other man." (Judges 16:17, KJV)

Not long after that, Samson was given a haircut, arrested, and, in an apocalyptic catastrophe, was killed along with his Philistine enemies.

Clearly this allegory was not intended to be a warning from God against hair loss, but many men today can relate to the visceral fear of the toll that *androgenetic alopecia* (genetic balding) can have on their virility.

If anything, the story of Samson and the collective anxiety that men and women share of going bald, illustrates how closely our hair is tied to our personal identities. Our hair, or lack thereof, is presumed, albeit unconsciously, to be a direct reflection of our personalities, our confidence, our sexual identities, and our outlook on life. Unfortunately, with today's emphasis on giving a good first impression in the job market and in the new realm of the online dating scene, this assumption has only gained in paramount importance.

Go to your favorite Internet search engine and type in the word "hair." The results will undoubtedly number in the tens of thousands, with the range of topics covering everything you can imagine: Chinese medicinal practices, how to find a good hair salon, conspiracy theories on the false cancer warnings of sodium laureth sulfate (a surfactant cleaning agent used in expensive salon shampoos), hundreds of websites and chat rooms dedicated to informing you about hair loss remedies, and even scores of sites dedicated to the classic rock musical *Hair*.

Admittedly, the quantity of information can be quite confusing, and perhaps more than a bit overwhelming. Added to that, many of those sites are really intended as promotions for expensive tonics, drugs, and products that promise startling results, but in most cases deliver disappointment and dangerous and unwelcome side effects—as well as a loud, annoying sucking sound as your money gets pulled down the drain.

This book is offered to you as an informative resource to answer your questions about hair care and give you a 7-Step Program to enhance your head of hair, whether or not you are battling hair loss. In the pages that follow, you will find a lot of information gleaned from nearly thirty years of hands-on research in the field of trichology. Included are many suggestions and methods for improving the health of your "crown of glory," while addressing the specific requirements of your particular hair type. Some of this may seem like common sense, but much of it will be quite surprising.

Most people have a visceral response to their own hair loss or damage that incorporates the belief that the problem must be localized somewhere between the follicle and the ends of their hair. Or they say, "That's just the way it is, so I guess I'll have to live with it." Those conclusions, while completely understandable, are frankly an erroneous outcome of deductive reasoning, or resigned frustration and tolerance. In the pages that follow, you will discover that the condition of your hair and scalp is a direct manifestation of what is going on throughout your body This book will not only offer healthy, viable, prudent solutions to your own particular condition by exploring alternatives to caring for your hair and scalp, but will also inquire into the role of exercise, diet, massage techniques, and skin care in maintaining a healthy head of hair.

We'll also take a look at the predominant causes of hair loss, debunk some of the ubiquitous myths of male pattern baldness (MPB), and suggest several effective and alternative methods for halting the progress of hair loss without the risk of surgery or uncertain prescription drugs and chemicals. You will also find a remarkably effective, comprehensive program—easily adaptable to your specific hair type and needs—that will stimulate the scalp to restore any remaining peach fuzz to its former full and healthy condition. If you're someone who is not suffering from this painful condition, you may be tempted to skip over those sections. *Don't.* The information, principles, and guidance will almost certainly be of value to you, and will expand your awareness of how hair works and how the body performs in generating a healthy scalp.

The advice offered in these pages is simple, practical, inexpensive, and safe, having been tested over and over again with thousands of people. Included are many recipes for hair and skin cleansers, scalp stimulators, astringents, and formulas for exfoliating dead tissue and unwanted particles that clog the follicles, effectively stunting the vitality of your hair—all of which you can prepare right in your own kitchen with ingredients you probably already have in your cupboards and refrigerator. If you don't know how to cook, don't worry. The recipes are about as complicated as boiling water and stirring with a spoon. *(A word to the wise: before including any of the formulas and recipes presented in these pages as part of your regular daily routine, it is suggested that you test them in small amounts to make certain there is no allergic reaction.)*

When you were born, you had the capacity to live your entire life with a full head of healthy, attractive hair. This book is intended to guide you so that you can realize that capacity. While much of the material may appear to be aimed specifically at people who are losing hair or going bald, it is really intended for everyone. The principals explored in the care of your scalp—hair care, skin care, diet, nutrition, exercise, and mind-body techniques—are applicable to anyone interested in having a healthy, full head of hair or anyone interested in restoring their crown of glory.

There is one caveat to those who are experiencing a condition of balding: if the hair follicles have completely stopped producing hair, *this is not something that can be reversed.* No one, not even the purveyors of Rogaine or Minoxidil, can change this. However, the program described in these pages will stop the *progression* of baldness. And wherever you can still feel the peach fuzz, there is hope. By rigorously following this program, your peach fuzz can be returned to its full, healthy, natural state. This unconventional, yet pragmatic approach toward altering your hair by altering your relationship to your body takes into account the interdependence of how you care for your hair, what you put into your body, and the consequences of your current lifestyle.

First things first, though. Let's take a look at hair, discover what it is, and examine some of the common reasons for hair loss and other associated problems.

2

How Hair Works:

A Basic Course in Trichology

As Francis Bacon once said, "Knowledge is power." Most people really know very little about how their bodies work, usually deferring this knowledge to a need-to-know basis when a medical crisis arises. Certainly this holds true when it comes to hair. If you're like the average Joe or Jane, you're probably quite content to wash it, comb it, and style it without ever giving a thought to what "it" actually is, or how it functions—until the day a friend gives you a snapshot they took of you at a recent party, or you look in the mirror and realize there's more hair in the washroom basin than on your scalp.

While you may be tempted to skip ahead to find out how to stop that receding hairline or repair those split ends, *don't do it*. This chapter will provide you with some critical and fundamental information about the structure of hair, and will be the basis for much of what is contained in the pages that follow. A little knowledge in the discipline of trichology, the study of hair and roots, will empower you to make informed and sensible decisions about your specific condition, allowing you to get the most out of the advice offered in these pages.

Upon close examination of the human body, you'll notice that virtually every part is adorned with hair. The only areas that are not covered are the lips, parts of the genitalia, soles of the feet, nipples, and palms of the hands. In fact, the human body contains more hair follicles per square inch on the surface of the skin than do most other primates in the animal kingdom. You might think that monkeys and apes are hairier, but this is a fallacy. Monkeys and apes simply have hair that is coarser and longer, but they don't have *more* hair.

We have two general types of hair: *vellus* hair that is extremely fine, and in many parts of the skin is virtually invisible to the naked eye. The second, more noticeable type, is classified as *terminal*, which can be found on the head, eyelids, face, pubic area, armpits, and on the chests of males.

The terminal fibers on the scalp are distinguishable by a set of different sub-types. The hairline begins from the base of the neck with a very fine fringe of terminal hairs that surround the circumference of the head, giving a subtle progression from the vellus fibers of the supposedly "bare" skin to the thicker terminal hairs adorning the crown.

Each hair shaft stems from a tiny gland under the epidermis called the *sebaceous gland*. The sebaceous gland produces a yellow, fatty secretion called *sebum*, which acts as a lubricant for the hair. (Sebum is the substance that causes oily skin and thus is a contributing factor in the formation of acne.) The hair shaft and sebaceous gland are surrounded by tiny *erector pili* muscles, which connect the base of the hair shaft to the underside of the skin. These erector pili muscles contract, effectively squeezing the sebaceous gland and causing the gland to lubricate the hair with sebum. (You probably have felt the erector pili muscles in your arms contract when someone has told you a good ghost story, or you've gotten goose pimples from a winter chill.)

The skin from which our hair arises is comprised of three distinct layers, the *epidermis*, the *dermis*, and *a layer of subcutaneous fat and connective tissue*.

The epidermis is composed of dead skin cells, and is generally about one millimeter in depth. The dead cells are in a constant state of sloughing, being replaced by newer dead cells when they fall off.

The second layer, the dermis, is roughly two to three millimeters thick on your scalp. This tough layer of connective tissue is where the sebaceous glands are located.

Below the dermis is more connective tissue, accompanied by a layer of subcutaneous fat. The blood vessels that nourish the skin are nestled here amongst millions of sensory nerve branches. On the scalp, this is the layer in which you will find the bulbous terminal hair follicles numbering from 100,000 to 150,000 on average. Each hair follicle measures three to four millimeters in length, and, just like the skin, has three layers: the pore from which the hair emanates, the *inner root sheath*, and the *cuticle*. This cuticle is the apparatus by which the hair shaft is held to the scalp.

At the base of the follicle is a tiny organ called the *papilla*, which extends up through the center of the follicle to the bottom of the hair. The papilla is what actually produces hair cells. A healthy papilla will become engorged with blood, from which it synthesizes proteins and formulates keratin, a protein comprised of a combination of carbon, hydrogen, nitrogen, sulfur, and oxygen. This protein forms 97 percent of the hair cells, which are forced up through the follicle, pushing up the older cells until they emerge from the scalp as your hair growth. The remaining 3 percent of the shaft is made up of amino acids, minerals, and a few other trace elements.

The hair shaft itself is *also* comprised of three layers of cells. The outermost layer, called the *cuticle*, is composed of complex, interlocking scalelike cells. These cells can be chemically stimulated to be raised, allowing for the absorption of moisture. This is in fact what happens when you use a conditioner, or have your hair colored, bleached, straightened, or curled. When hair is referred to as "damaged," the cuticle layer is where most of this "damage" has occurred.

The cells of the *cortex*, the second layer of the hair shaft, are elongated, providing strength and flexibility. The cortex also contains the pigmentation, which gives the hair its natural color.

The round cells of the third layer, the *medulla*, are the marrow of the hair shaft and are frequently not found in hair that is very fine.

Hair grows in stages. At any given moment, about 90 percent of the terminal hairs on your scalp are presently growing at a rate of about a half-inch per month. These hairs are in the *anagen* stage, a period which commonly lasts from two to seven years. The remaining 10 percent are in a dormant state called *telogen*, which normally lasts for about three months. During this resting phase, the papilla stops producing keratin and the hair shaft detaches from the gland, eventually falling away from the scalp. A new hair will take its place when the papilla returns to the anagen stage.

When the growth cycles from anagen to telogen to anagen again are functioning properly, most people should lose an average of eighty to one hundred hairs per day. Anything more than that indicates that something is awry.

Which brings us to the end of our introductory course in trichology. Now that you have a basic understanding of the physiology of hair and how it works, let's turn to the more advanced topics of the causes of hair loss and other common issues.

3

The Causes of Hair Loss and Other Problems:

An Advanced Course in Trichology

With a rudimentary understanding of the physiology of hair behind us, we can now begin to turn our attention to the subject that is the concern of so many men and women, and is probably one of the primary reasons you're holding this book right now: hair loss.

Before we can begin to address the solutions to this all-too-common affliction, an understanding of the fundamental types of hair loss and their causes will be crucial to the implementation of any successful hair restoration program.

To reiterate, losing hair is normal. Most people lose between eighty to one hundred terminal hairs per day from their scalp. This is even true of the majority of people who are experiencing hair loss or thinning, known as *alopecia* ("al-oh-pee-sha"). When the follicles of people suffering from alopecia shift into the dormant telogen period, the hair falls out at the same rate as healthy people. The difference is that the follicle closes up and shuts down rather than reawakening to the active anagen stage. There are some types of alopecia that result in elevated rates of shedding, often losing whole clumps of hair at a time, but this condition is rare and we'll discuss this in further detail a bit later.

There are several classifications of alopecia, with the most prevalent being *androgenetic alopecia*, the culprit in over 95 percent of hair loss cases. Both men and women experience androgenetic alopecia. For men, it is often pronounced and dishearteningly visible for all the world to see, and is commonly referred to as male pattern baldness (MPB). In women, it is usually fairly diffuse, occurring over broader regions of the scalp, resulting in an overall thinning of the hair rather than the development of any discernible pattern of baldness.

Androgenetic alopecia is widely recognized as a genetic trait passed down from either parent. This is why it is known as "pattern" baldness, since the same patterns tend to show up throughout the family tree. The genetic code for hair loss sends hormone messages to the cells in the follicles associated with the family pattern. The hormone messages essentially tell the papilla in these follicles to grow thinner and less hair, eventually shutting them down until they grow no hair at all.

Those hormones that direct the hair follicles are part of an extensive assortment of hormones called *androgens*. Testosterone, an androgen that is present in men and women, plays an essential role in the genetic code's mandate for pattern hair loss. Hormone levels deviate from person to person, and fluctuate at different stages in their life.

As the blood carries testosterone to the hair follicle, it interacts with an enzyme called 5-alpha reductase, converting the hormone into dihydrotestosterone (DHT). DHT restricts the vasodilation (blood flow) to the papilla at the base of the follicle. In short, it is the culprit that provokes hair loss, hence androgenetic alopecia.

Estrogen obstructs the effects of DHT. Since women have higher levels of estrogen than men do, most women are safeguarded from androgenetic alopecia—that is, until they reach menopause, when the levels of estrogen take a sudden, sharp drop in the bloodstream. With the DHT newly unimpeded, the onset of hair thinning in menopausal women can sometimes be quite dramatic in its rapidity.

Before losing heart, there is one other important factor to keep in mind: the genetic code merely determines a *tendency* toward DHT's vasodilation of the papilla. If unchecked, hair loss will certainly result. However, there are many methods for interrupting this process, and we'll explore some of them in the next chapter.

Another form of hair loss is *traction alopecia*, which occurs when the hair shafts are subjected to the constant pulling of tightly braided hairstyles, plucking, tweezing, and waxing. This traumatizes the follicles and leads to the hairs falling out before the completion of their growth cycle. Usually traction alopecia is temporary, taking three to four months for the follicles to recover. Nonetheless, repeatedly subjecting the same follicles to this constant pulling will eventually lead to permanent hair loss.

About one percent of the population suffers from a condition called *alopecia areata*, an autoimmune condition in which the white blood cells interpret the hair follicles as an invading tissue that must be expelled from the body. Alopecia areata customarily causes people to lose hair on the scalp in smooth, circular clumps typically about one inch in diameter. In severe cases this can expand to the loss of all scalp hair (*alopecia totalis*), and sometimes expands to the loss of all hair on the body (*alopecia universalis*). Typically, this incurable autoimmune complication is temporary, although its duration is entirely unpredictable.

Telogen effluvium is a form of hair loss resulting from sudden, severe stress. This can be a rather traumatic occurrence because the shedding of hair is always delayed, in most cases three to four months and sometimes as much as six months *after* the originating stressful event (*i.e.*, a job termination, divorce, or death of a loved one). Telogen effluvium strikes randomly across the scalp, and is most often noticeable only to the person suffering from the infliction. It is temporary, since there has been no damage to the follicle. Most of the hairs will return once the normal anagen and telogen growth cycles resume.

Childbirth can provoke telogen effluvium, but not because it is a stressful event (which it certainly can be for many women). It's really triggered by sudden changes in hormones after giving birth. During pregnancy, estrogen levels surge sufficiently to inhibit the dormant telogen period in a considerable percentage of the scalp. This is why pregnant women notice that their hair seems fuller. It is because there are more active follicles growing hair. Immediately following childbirth, those follicles that usually would have been dormant suddenly get the message that it's time for a rest. Within a few months some new mothers will begin to shed hair, sometimes in distressing quantities.

Pregnancy terminations, abortions, and miscarriages can also result in telogen effluvium if enough of the woman's hair follicles have missed their telogen period.

Discontinuing the use of certain contraceptive pills sometimes has the side effect of triggering telogen effluvium, since many of these drugs operate by adding hormones to the woman's bloodstream. Essentially, they work by fooling the reproductive system into thinking the woman is already pregnant, thus raising the estrogen levels and further inhibiting the telogen period. Once the dosage of the drug is stopped, the normal growth cycles kick in and there is the resultant telogen effluvium.

Anagen effluvium is the abrupt loss of hair from the chemicals and radiation treatments prescribed for cancer patients. Quite the opposite of telogen effluvium, where the hair loss begins after three or four months, the hair loss of anagen effluvium commences within one to three weeks after a treatment. These patients can expect that either some or all of their hair will fall out. Chemotherapy and radiation therapy work by killing the rapidly dividing cells characteristic of cancer. Unfortunately, the treatment also kills other rapidly dividing cells, such as the ones being produced by the papilla in the hair follicles. In most cases, this condition is temporary, and within six months to a year the hair will begin to regrow.

Nutritional deficiencies play a large factor in hair loss and health. The human body is essentially comprised of three basic types of tissues: carbohydrates, fats, and proteins. Remembering that the hair shaft is made up of 97 percent protein, it is useful to realize that the processes for synthesizing proteins requires a great deal more energy than that of carbohydrates and fats. When a person is malnourished or ill, the hair stops growing and the hair shafts will begin to look less and less healthy. The condition of the hair is a direct manifestation of a person's health.

Hair shaft breakage (damage to the hair itself) can also result in hair loss. Several things can cause breakage. One of the worst offenses is the use of hairstyling chemicals, particularly the inexpensive isopropyl alcohol-based gels, sprays, and mousses you can find at just about any supermarket, drug store, or discount store. Hair dyes, bleaches, relaxers (straighteners most frequently used by African-Americans), and permanent wave solutions can wreak a lot of damage, especially if you use them with any regularity.

Blow-dryers and curling irons can make the hair shaft highly prone to breakage. Excessive heat causes the shafts to become weak and brittle.

Improper grooming techniques cause damage, as well. Using a comb or brush when your hair is wet and at its weakest should never be done. In fact, never use a brush on wet hair. Use a wide-toothed comb or your fingers! (More about brushes later.)

Men who part their hair are particularly susceptible to hair loss. Parting the hair, which is usually done with a comb while the hair is wet, causes a weakening of the follicles and hair shafts in the crown where the hair is combed. Again, the use of a wide-toothed comb—or better yet, your fingers—is strongly urged.

Excessive shampooing with inexpensive store-bought products can dry out your hair, making it brittle and prone to breakage. The same can be said for vigorous shampooing, improper scalp massage, or towel-drying techniques.

Chlorine and sunlight weaken the hair shafts, too. When swimming, you should cover your scalp with a swimming cap to avoid exposure. If you don't like the idea of a swimming cap, then wash your hair immediately upon leaving the pool or ocean. When going out into the bright sunlight, wearing a hat will block the damaging rays of the sun.

Perhaps the most important factor in hair loss is how almost every single one of the conditions described here affect the sebaceous gland and it secretion of the lubricating sebum. What happens 99 percent of the time (particularly in MPB), whether the papilla's production of keratin is disrupted by the genetic balding messages carried in DHT or the hair shaft has suffered breakage from too much bleaching, sebum begins to build up in the follicle. The follicle then becomes blocked, inducing further damage to the tiny structure and effectively cutting off any chances for the hair to survive. This, in fact, is the literal root cause of hair loss.

Now let's turn to perhaps the most controversial section of this book: the various methods prevalently employed to restore hair by treating the conditions and symptoms described in this chapter.

4

How to Earn $7 Billion a Year:

The Business of Hair Loss

mhotep, a royal priest who lived 4,000 years ago in the Old Kingdom of the Nile Valley, is regarded as the architect who originated the iconic design of the pyramids of Ancient Egypt. He is also commonly acknowledged as the Father of Medicine, with numerous unearthed medical papyrus texts being attributed to him. The Edwin Smith Surgical Papyrus, which is among the oldest writings ever discovered, has been dated at around 1700 BC, and is particularly noteworthy for encapsulating Imhotep's remarkable clinical precision.

Sadly, his keen sense of observation, empiricism, and no-nonsense results has not always been the keystone for the discipline of medicine. This has been particularly so for the practice of hair restoration. Indeed, even in Imhotep's own kingdom one can find such ludicrous prescriptions as a compound constituted from the dung of a hippopotamus with liberal dollops of crocodile fat in equal parts, which was then applied directly to the scalp. Almost a thousand years later, Hippocrates, who fostered the enduring medical ethic known as the Hippocratic Oath, refined his Egyptian predecessor's prescription with a recipe calling for cumin, horseradish, nettles, and fresh pigeon droppings.

Things have improved only slightly over the ages, with many senseless (and even downright dangerous) methods and tonics being passed off as remedies for hair loss. Today, the search for a cure has ballooned to an industry with estimated annual earnings in excess of $7 billion. To make matters worse, much of the industry is cloaked in the credible mantle of scientific research, funded by large drug manufacturers with slick and comforting ad campaigns churned out by executive committees in glass towers lining the New York skyline along Madison Avenue. Frankly, they're not too far removed from the snake-oil salesmen slithering through the frontiers of the Old West.

What these massive pharmaceutical and surgical corporations are not willing to state up front in their glossy print ads and cozy prime-time, thirty-second spots is this: they don't have a cure. They don't even understand for certain why DHT shuts down keratin production in the papilla. In effect, all they are selling is a treatment for the *symptoms* by fending off the inevitable progression of further hair loss. And if you ever stop using their drugs or don't check in for additional surgery, your condition will regress to the way it was before you started, often rapidly degenerating to a worsened predicament.

To put it bluntly, the only guarantee they can offer with impunity is that your bank account will be seeing a lot more red ink.

Currently the Food and Drug Administration (FDA) has approved only two drugs for wide use in the United States:

minoxidil, commonly sold under the registered trademark name Rogaine, and finasteride, a daily pill marketed as Propecia.

Minoxidil was originally introduced as a treatment for high blood pressure. This drug is prescribed for hypertensive patients only as a last resort, since it is known to have some very severe side effects: chiefly chronic fluid retention, which eventually results in congestive heart failure.

Another less threatening side effect became apparent shortly after it was introduced: patients began growing hair in some pretty peculiar places, such as the backs of their hands and their foreheads. After an intuitive leap of logic and more testing in the Upjohn science labs, it turned out that minoxidil regrew hair when applied as a topical cream on the partially balding scalps of men with none of the life-threatening side effects of the oral version.

It does not work on areas of the scalp that are completely bald, where the follicles have died. Neither does it appear to have any regrowth effects on the front part of the scalp. Furthermore, minoxidil's restorative properties appear to be temporary at best. Eventually, the DHT levels in the bloodstream build up a resistance and overpower any benefits the drug bestows. In time, the patient will resume going bald.

Other problems include the fact that results are frequently not visible for at least six to twelve months—and that's only if it's applied twice a day *without fail*. Additionally, minoxidil has difficulties being absorbed into the follicles of the scalp, so it is frequently manufactured with Retin-A, a topical retinoic acid that acts as a conductive agent. Retin-A increases the absorption levels of minoxidil, but it too has side effects. It commonly causes skin irritation, rashes, infection, and scarring, all of which—ironically enough—lead to permanent hair loss.

Finasteride, manufactured by Merck under the trademark Propecia, is only somewhat of an improvement over minoxidil. Originally, it was designed to treat benign prostate hyperplasia, and, like minoxidil, it too had the unexpected side effect of inducing hair growth. Merck's science team discovered that cutting the prostate medication to a one-fifth dosage was sufficient for the treatment of hair loss. Since it is a pill taken once a day rather than a cream applied twice a day, it's easier to manage the dosages.

Following the adage that less is more, however, Propecia costs two to four times the price of Rogaine.

That's not the only side effect, either.

Impotence, diminished libido, and a decreased volume of ejaculate are experienced in some men, as well as gynecomastia, an enlargement of the breasts. (Although women may think this might be a desirable side effect worth obtaining a prescription for, it should be noted that this condition occurs only in men.) Propecia also lowers prostate specific antigens (PSA) in the bloodstream, making it extremely difficult for the detection of prostate cancer. Women of childbearing years should not touch any crushed tablets of the drug with their bare fingers or skin, as it is also known to cause severe birth defects.

The good news is that most of the side effects will disappear within a few weeks after discontinuing the use of Propecia. The bad news is that you'll lose all the hair you regrew within two to six months. So once you've started using Propecia, *you can never stop*.

Moreover, the FDA, which was commissioned with the responsibility of determining the safety and effectiveness of medications distributed in the United States, uncharacteristically approved Propecia *without the benefit of any long-term studies on its effectiveness*. (In fact, it certainly appears that the potential revenue that would eventually be earned by Merck persuasively eclipsed any reasonable scientific methodology the FDA applied in its decision-making process.) No one knows if the DHTs in the bloodstream will build up a resistance, like minoxidil, and overpower the drug. It's simply too early to tell.

Currently, there are several other potential drugs in various testing stages with the FDA, some of which are intended for prescription use by women. Without exception, though, these newer drugs do have side effects ranging from a mild and reversible reduction of testosterone levels in men and progesterone in women, to toxic, irreversible damage to the liver.

Surgical treatments for hair loss have enjoyed a surge in popularity, and the consequent leap in profits, due to vast improvements in technology over the last ten years. Though hair restoration specialists can now be found in virtually every medical clinic around the corner, the results have not improved by much.

Slick advertising is used to sell the idea that surgery is now the answer to hair restoration. This is a blatant canard to state it mildly. No new hair is added to the scalp. It's simply moved from the areas that aren't (apparently) programmed for androgenetic alopecia, giving the *illusion* of more hair. Be it a micrograft, full-sized hair plug, scalp lift, or reduction, *it does not stop hair loss. Period.*

For surgery to produce convincing results, it typically requires several procedures, each of which must be administered three to four months apart. Each procedure can cost anywhere from several hundred dollars to several thousand. Most insurance companies categorize hair restoration as an elective procedure and therefore do not pay out any benefits; so most patients must finance the surgery with credit cards or a second mortgage. (Oddly enough, one of the selling points of surgery is that it supposedly costs less than drug treatments spread out over a lifetime.)

The use of laser technology has been heavily promoted in recent years with assurances of less time in the operating room and reduced cosmetic complications such as scarring, bumps, or depressions that commonly result from the old-style metal instruments. But lasers are an expensive investment, which has assuredly tempted many a surgeon to aggrandize their benefits in an attempt to pay them off. The cost of the hardware is passed on to the patient.

The surgeon rarely passes on complete information to the patient about the vital drawbacks of laser surgery that might cause a patient to seek assistance elsewhere: the laser burns a tiny hole in the scalp where the redistributed hair follicle is to be placed. The hole is very precise, which is the major selling point of laser surgery. This hole is supposed to heal faster and cleaner than the holes made from old-style metal instruments. Nevertheless, because the burst of light must be quite intense, it often burns additional cells immediately surrounding the hole. This slows the natural fibrin bonding process, which is the first stage of healing when a new follicle is inserted. The follicle takes longer to reconnect to the blood supply, increasing the risk of a lower yield of hair growth.

Essentially, the patient has paid for a really expensive light show.

Artificial hair transplants are available in Japan and some European countries. Although recent developments have produced extremely realistic synthetic hairs that produce marvelous and immediate cosmetic results, there are some serious drawbacks. The FDA has banned this procedure since 1984 because in every single case, the body's immune system eventually rejects the synthetic hairs as a foreign substance. Often, chronic inflammation and bacterial infections in the scalp accompany the immune response, leading to infection of living hair follicles and increased hair loss.

Doctors in Japan, Mexico, and a few European countries also offer a surgical procedure for attaching a hairpiece that can be removed for ease of cleaning. The hairpiece is attached most commonly with osseointegrated pins. These pins are made of titanium and are permanently imbedded into the skull. Bone tissue grows around the pins over time, fastening them securely. The hairpiece, which looks very realistic, is fitted with metal snaps that attach to the pins. The only problem with this procedure is that it is *extremely* dangerous. Any operation that entails cutting into the skull is considered risky. Leaving a foreign object in the skull, even surgical-grade titanium, which is exposed to the outside environment of the scalp, is playing with rather dicey odds stacked in favor of a lethal brain infection. The surgery required to remove the pins is even more dangerous than implanting them.

Seven billion dollars a year is generated in the United States alone by the treatments described here. Not one of them actually addresses the source of the problem, attacking it from only one narrow viewpoint, or, as in the case of surgery, avoiding a genuine solution altogether. The human body is a complex machine, with all of its parts elegantly integrated into a wondrous whole.

When viewed as a wondrous whole, a solution does in fact present itself. A solution that is in perfect alignment with the natural processes of the human organism, and improves not just the health of the scalp, but also the well-being of the entire body. As we said in the previous chapter, the body is comprised of carbohydrates, fats, and proteins, with hair being 97 percent protein. The condition of the hair is a direct reflection of the condition of the whole body. Simple intuitive logic argues that a program that addresses hair care from a holistic perspective will obtain results that permanently interrupt further hair loss and improve the condition of the hair, the overall health of the body, and the quality of life.

This holistic perspective is one that pharmaceutical and surgical companies have ignored and derided in the interest of elevated profits. What follows in the remaining sections of this book is a program that will empower you with a solution that will actually get to the root—so to speak—of the problem, and won't require a second mortgage on your house.

It will require an unerring level of rigor. The program, once begun, must be followed *exactly* as prescribed. Any deviance from the program will disrupt the process, and you will have to start again. The program will also require a transformation in thought. There will be ideas and techniques that will challenge your thinking, sounding rather fantastic and unusual. Trust must be the key word here. The program has been tested and refined on thousands of clients over the past thirty years. Every one of them would tell you the same thing: "The program works."

It will also require a transformation in lifestyle. You will discover that there are certain practices that you currently have in your life which don't support your health, and more directly don't support the health of your hair. The program suggests simple ways to alter or remove these practices, while greatly improving your quality of life.

So, take a deep breath, and let's begin.

5

Before You Get Started:

Set Yourself Up for Success

In this chapter, I'm going to get you ready to begin. First, you're going to start with a clean slate, then you're going to begin to record your progress, and finally, you're going to lay the groundwork for a holistic approach to a new head of hair.

Start with a Clean Slate

Before you begin the program, there's one big thing you have to do...

Go to your bathroom. Collect all of your hair care products: your shampoos, conditioners, gels, mousses, sprays, relaxers, dyes, everything. Including the expensive products your stylist sold you during your last trip to the salon.

Now throw them away.

Yes, that's right. *Throw them away.* (Or rather, rinse them out and recycle the containers.) Those over-the-counter items are another one of the causes of hair damage and loss.

Take a look at the ingredients label on your favorite bottle of shampoo before you toss it in the recycling bin. Whatever is shown first on the list is what there is the most of in the bottle, and what comes at the end of the list is what's least. The first ingredient will almost certainly be water ("eau," if the manufacturer's marketing department has settled on building the snob appeal by including a French translation). Second or third on the list will be a chemical surfactant, which is intended to help the cleaning agents lather more, or it could also be the primary cleaning agent. The two common surfactants used in shampoos are *ammonium laurel sulfate* and *sodium laureth (or laurel) sulfate*. Ammonium laurel sulfate is used in most cheap or inexpensive shampoos from your drug store or grocery. Sodium laureth sulfate, which is gentler, is used in most salon products, and is the primary reason they are more expensive than your drug store shampoo. The salon products also probably include one or two high-quality protein conditioners, which also accounts for their higher cost.

The remaining ingredients on the label are intended as preservatives or for consumer appeal: a pleasant color to the shampoo, aroma, and whatever the latest buzzword is in the marketing world, like aloe, honey, or the current herbal scent. (Yes, honey and herbs are wonderful ingredients to use on your hair, but not in the minimal quantities used in a shampoo purchased from a store or salon. Aloe can also be good, too, but only if it is stabilized aloe. Otherwise it's just a clever way of selling more water.)

Many of these over-the-counter shampoos and conditioners leave a heavy silicon-like deposit under the cuticle of the hair shaft. Eventually, it leaves enough deposits to cause breakage, and is the reason most people feel they have to change shampoos every few months.

For those of you who use a dandruff shampoo, throw that away, too (unless you have a prescription from your doctor). You have been duped by the shampoo industry into believing you have dandruff. Most likely you don't. Almost nobody actually has dandruff. The industry marketing departments have done a stellar job of selling the idea that a flaking scalp is caused by dandruff. It's not! The only cause of flaking is having a dry scalp. Dandruff is a rare condition of oily, yellow, or gray powder clumping together to form tiny balls—never flakes. Once you start on the program, your flaking scalp will be healed very quickly, so throw that bottle away immediately.

Now you will need something to replace all of those products. With each of the seven steps, I'll give you recipes for shampoos, rinses, conditioners, and styling gels that are 100 percent natural, can be made right in your kitchen, and can be readily adjusted for the specific needs of each member of your family. If you don't know how to cook, don't worry. Pretty much all you need to know how to do is boil water, and to do a little stirring and mixing. That's it.

You will also need to take a trip to the supermarket or health food store. At the end of this book, you'll find some additional information about plants and herbs that will help you in your shopping. You may find that buying all of the ingredients at the start of the program may seem like a considerable expense initially, but most of the recipes are extremely concentrated. In a very short time, you will see that you're saving a substantial amount over the cost of the hair care products and restoratives you were buying before.

Record Your Progress

One more thing before we go any further—it's time to take a snapshot of where you're at right now. Literally.

When working with clients on the program, it is always best to begin by taking photographs so they can clearly see their progress over time. This is particularly important for keeping them grounded in reality. Over the course of the 90 days, as you implement the life changes necessary for the transformation of your scalp, you will go through a lot of stages. You'll probably start out the program with a heightened sense of gusto and commitment. Then one day you'll wake up and wonder what the heck you're doing, and mutter at your reflection in the mirror, "What's the point? It's taking too long! I'm wasting my time!"

It's at moments like that where's it's very useful to pull out your photos to see where you were when you started on Day One. There's nothing like a good dose of reality to jolt you out of the doldrums when you see that you've actually made a great deal of progress in a relatively short period of time. You will clearly see that all your hard work, dedication, commitment, and integrity have indeed been paying off. These photographs are a record of your success.

The camera doesn't lie. Having a clear, impartial measurement for your success like a photograph is an extremely useful tool for keeping on track and sticking with the program. Many clients over the years have attested to this, and have been thankful for the pictures.

These aren't portraits you'll be taking, so either a Polaroid or a digital camera will do. You'll also need a well-lit room and a willing assistant to take the pictures.

1. Start by having your partner take a photo of your face from about the shoulder up. Be sure to leave room at the top of the frame for your entire scalp.
2. Next, take a shot of the right profile, making sure that the entire scalp is visible.
3. Repeat Step 2 for the left profile.
4. Take a shot of the back of your head from the shoulders up.
5. Finally, your partner needs to get a shot of the top of your head. You can cither lean over by dropping your chin to your chest, or you can kneel on the floor.

In every shot, make certain your partner can clearly see the damage or areas of hair loss and thinning through the lens. If you can't see it when you print it out or get it developed, then it won't be much use as a measurement of your success.

If your camera does not indicate the date on the prints, you need to date them yourself. Place the photographs in a small album, or glue them into a notebook. You'll be adding a new set of pictures at the end of three months, and then every three months after that, so get out your calendar and schedule your photography sessions for the next twelve months. After the first 90 days, you will most likely already see a startling difference.

6

The 7-Step Program:

What You Can Expect

As we have seen in the previous chapter, merely attacking the symptoms of hair loss or damage really does nothing to resolve the condition. In fact, what is required is nothing short of a full-body transformation. A healthy, functioning body is tantamount to generating a healthy head of hair. If that sounds like a lot of work, it really isn't. Affecting a full-fledged transformation does not necessarily require a huge effort. For most people the hardest part will be the effort to maintain vigilance and rigor in sticking to the program. *You must follow every step and every recipe, every day for the next 90 days.*

Is it difficult? No.

The 7-Step Program that follows is actually very simple. All of the techniques and tips can be incorporated into your daily routine with a great deal of ease. Many suggestions are included to assist you in making the program an ordinary part of your day-to-day life.

As reinforcement for your commitment, it is strongly recommended that you invite your spouse, children, or life-partner to participate in the program with you. Change is always easiest when you have the full support of those closest to you. Since the program is designed to promote vitality and health throughout the whole body, they will assuredly reap benefits just as extraordinary as your own healthy head of hair. Included are many variations and much information specifically addressing the needs of each member of your family, whether they are suffering from a form of alopecia, split ends, or simply want to enhance the condition of their hair.

The results of this 7-Step Program may be almost immediate. As new sets of follicles awaken from the dormant telogen state, many people who follow this program will see voluminous, healthy hair shafts from the very first week. For others, it will take a little longer. In all cases, the full impact will continue to be seen for up to 52 weeks. After all, the time to build up to your current condition of hair loss or damage probably took many years longer to develop.

But there is so much more than that. As we pointed out in Chapter One, your hair is closely connected to your identity and to how you feel about yourself. As you begin to see results, you will start to notice a transformation in your state of being, in your self-esteem. Your success cannot help but boost your sense of well-being, joy, dignity, and confidence. As you implement these suggested modifications to your lifestyle, you will begin to see extraordinary changes in how you feel about yourself. This program, time-tested with thousands of clients over thirty years, represents nothing less than the dawning of a whole new unrecognizable you.

Step One: The Magic Haircut

A haircut, you say, has nothing to do with hair growth. Ordinarily this is correct, but when you are talking about turning peach fuzz on a balding head into healthy, thriving hair, it is quite a different story.

As I have explained, much of your hair loss can be attributed to the condition of your scalp. Waxy buildup and dead cells form a barrier that quite literally asphyxiates the roots of this baby-fine hair. Once this life-source has been smothered, your hair cannot grow.

Those silky fine hairs that you can feel when you run your fingers through your hair—that peach fuzz we have been talking about—cannot survive and grow into strong, long-lasting hair if it has to struggle to get through a wall of wax and dead cells. The root will become so weakened from decreased blood flow (caused by the lack of nutrition) that it won't be strong enough to push through the pore.

The treatments in this program, as well as thorough brushing and proper massage, will dissolve the oils and waxes blocking the scalp and will remove anything that adheres to the scalp. They will also balance the condition of the hair and scalp, normalizing the hair's acid mantle and stabilizing the flow of the sebaceous glands that keep the scalp (and in turn, the hair) pliant and lubricated.

The right haircut—one that relieves any pressure on new hair as it emerges from below the scalp—is the foundation to the entire program.

I call it my Magic Cut because it works like a magic charm that helps your hair grow with ease. Take this book with you to your stylist, and show him/her these instructions:

1. The hairline must be cut with precision and care. Every single hair must be lifted with a comb and cut. Your stylist will comb a thin layer forward and clip, then section another layer forward and clip it even with the first, repeating the process until all hair has been sectioned and cut from the front hairline to the crown. Even if you do it yourself, have your hairline trimmed every three weeks. Just a tiny bit at the ends. Lift your hair with your comb and take tiny snips—even of the fuzz.

2. Once the horizontal layering of the top is complete, the same area must be layered and cut on an angle, vertically with the sides. Work from the front to the back on each side. Such careful distribution of the hair's volume creates a balanced, easily styled look for both men and women.

3. Working from the crown, your stylist will section your hair vertically in small sections. Lift hair and cut over the comb. Alternate cutting vertically with cutting horizontally until you reach the nape.

4. Be careful to integrate the layering from both sides and the crown so that you won't have a strong line across your head. Even fuzz must be combed and clipped to prohibit damage and drying as it grows.

5. Angular cutting at the sides strengthens and shapes hair at the temples. Regular cutting will enable your hair to grow

into shape. By the time you complete the 7-Step Program, the styling patterns of the basic Magic Cut will be established.

By carefully sectioning the hair and clipping the ends of each section horizontally and then resectioning so that it can be cut vertically, your stylist will be able to create "tunnels" through the under-layers of your hair. This technique provides "lift"—air space—from underneath so that your new hair will have room to grow. In this way, any weight that might press down on the peach fuzz that we are transforming into hair will be removed.

You will find that, as you use the scalp and hair treatments and your hair begins to grow stronger and healthier than ever before, you will need to have your hair cut more often.

I suggest that the clients who come into my clinic have a cut every three or four weeks instead of every two to three months.

This is a surprise to them at first, but within the first month of the program, they understand why I say this. Their hair is growing faster than ever.

The same cutting principles I've outlined for the Magic Cut on men should be used for women's hair or for longer hairstyles. In fact, if children have their hair cut this way from an early age, it can prevent later hair loss. Certainly, short hair is lighter in weight than long or even medium-length hair, but with the Magic Cut, this weight will not press down on new hair growth.

A client who has very fine but thick gray-blond hair swears by the Magic Cut because it adds volume to her relatively straight hair. As her hair is becoming gray, she has noticed that the gray hair is coarser than the blond and is slightly wavy in comparison to her super-straight ash-blond hair. The Magic Cut complements the texture of her hair, which, thanks to my regimen program, is healthier than it has been since she was a little girl with cornsilk hair.

Step Two: The Right Way to Brush Your Hair

The key to stimulating and retaining a healthful mane of hair is increasing and maintaining the quality and abundance of blood flow to the papilla in the hair follicles. If normal vasodilation (blood flow) is obstructed, either from the genetic messages engendered in androgenetic alopecia (MPB), stress (which causes telogen effluvium), or poor grooming habits inflaming and clogging the scalp follicles and sebaceous glands, vital nutrients and oxygen are cut off from the follicle. Without these nutrients and oxygen, the follicle dies. Hair will not grow.

Brushing your hair properly is an essential part of stimulating the blood flow to the hair follicles.

Your Hairbrush

But before we talk about brushing, let's take a look at your brush. Take a few moments, set this book down, and go to your bathroom to retrieve your brush. While you're at it, grab your comb. Don't forget the ones in your briefcase or purse as well.

Take a look at them. Now ask yourself, "When was the last time I washed this?" If you're like most people, you can't remember.

Think about this: every time you washed your hair to get it clean, you probably used your brush or comb to style it afterwards—the dirty brush or comb you're holding right now. Think about this, as well: isn't it a lot like taking a shower and putting on dirty clothes again?

All that collected dirt and oil just goes back onto your hair and scalp, effectively reclogging the pores and follicles you just cleansed with shampoo. You need to clean your brushes and combs *every day that you use them*. This can be done in the shower while you shampoo, since shampoo is the best product to clean them with. Shampoo is designed to remove the oils and dirt that collect on the scalp, and it works just as well on your brush.

Administer a small amount of shampoo onto the bristles, and work it into the brush. Run your comb through the bristles to loosen the dirt and oil. Rinse in hot water, and then repeat until thoroughly clean. Give it a good shake to release the excess water, then dry on a soft cloth towel. After the initial cleaning, it should be quite easy to maintain if practiced on a daily basis.

If you have no interest in taking the time to clean your brush, then you can wrap it in cheesecloth. The cheesecloth will not interfere with the bristles, and will collect the grime and oil from your hair. The cloth should be changed daily.

There are many types of brushes available, but the best kind is made from boar's hair. You can find this type at any beauty supply store or salon. The bristles are very similar to the keratin of human hair and absorb oil and dirt just like your hairs do. Nylon brushes do not work anywhere near as effectively as boar's hair, and are not recommended. Another benefit of natural bristles is that the tips of the bristles are rounded, which is gentler on the scalp and hair shafts. Nylon bristles are usually sharp, and can lead to follicle inflammation and hair breakage.

Brushes and combs should be replaced at least once a year. Eventually the bristles will weaken and break, which leads to split ends and breakage.

Brushing

Never use a brush when your hair is damp. Hair expands when it comes into contact with water, essentially weakening the outer cuticle layer and making the shaft noticeably brittle. The hair becomes so elastic when wet that brushing could easily stretch the shafts to the breaking point. Use a wide-toothed comb with rounded teeth.

A regimen of brushing (when your hair is dry) is a critical part of preventing hair loss and nurturing the vitality of your hair. The gentle pulling from brushing stimulates vasodilation to the scalp. It encourages the proper functioning of the tiny erector pili muscles to squeeze the sebaceous glands, which lubricates the hair with sebum, promoting a more lustrous, healthy condition. Additionally, brushing removes dead cells from the epidermis, dirt, and any remaining waxy buildup.

To succeed at stimulating the scalp, you must brush twice a day: once in the morning and again in the evening. Gently brush for three to five minutes (three minutes for short hair, five minutes for longer). If you bend your head to the floor, you will increase the amount of blood circulation, which will maximize the benefits of brushing. Brush from the neck forward to the front of the scalp, then from the sides to the crown of the scalp. Finally, brush from the front of the scalp toward the neck.

If your hair has tangles, work them out delicately from the ends.

Step Three: Stimulate the Scalp

For healthy, strong hair to grow, the scalp must be completely free of excess oils and dead cells, and the roots must be well fed. This means that blood must flow freely through the scalp. To accomplish this, you'll massage special oils into your scalp that are well known for their abilities to stimulate blood circulation as well as hair growth. *Do this every single night at bedtime, without fail.*

As you massage these fragrant, stimulating oils into your scalp, you will feel a tingling sensation. This is caused by the blood which is now circulating through your scalp like never before. It is important that you massage your forehead and neck as well as your scalp. Make sure that the oils actually penetrate your skin. They have important work to do!

You will use a Daytime Scalp Stimulator in the morning and Nighttime Scalp Stimulator nightly, and a Super Scalp Stimulator, applied once a week. Here are the recipes:

Daytime Scalp Stimulator

APPLY EVERY MORNING

3 ounces cayenne pepper

A fifth of vodka

Combine the cayenne pepper with the vodka and let stand for fifteen days. Shake daily. Strain, pour into a bottle with a cap, and label.

Rub into the scalp every morning, being sure to keep away from the eyes, then brush and style the hair. If you have bleached or light hair, test on a small strand of hair before applying to your entire head.

Alternative (nonalcoholic) Daytime Scalp Stimulator

Mix equal parts of castor oil and white iodine

(both may be purchased at a pharmacy)

Store in a labeled squeeze bottle. Shake before using.

Rub into the scalp in the morning, then brush and style the hair.

Nighttime Scalp Stimulator

APPLY EVERY NIGHT

6 teaspoons rosemary oil

3 teaspoons basil oil (if available; otherwise use

2 teaspoons rosemary oil)

3 teaspoons lavender oil

2 teaspoons lemon oil

Put the oils into an amber glass bottle with a glass dropper

top. Close tightly and shake well to mix. Label.

Pour two teaspoons of Nighttime Scalp Stimulator into a glass bowl. Massage into your scalp with your fingertips. Divide your hair into small sections at the hairline and work from the forehead to the crown. Concentrate on the areas of balding, then distribute the remainder over the rest of your head, hairline, and ends of hair.

Leave the Nighttime Scalp Stimulator on your head overnight. Most of the oils will have been absorbed by your hair and scalp, so you need not be concerned about getting oil on your pillow. But if you want to play it safe, cover your pillow with a terry cloth towel.

In the morning, wash out with the Hair and Scalp Shampoo (see pages 57–58).

If you suffer from dandruff, here is a Scalp Stimulator that relieves dandruff. Use it in place of the Nighttime Scalp Stimulator one to three times per week.

Alternative Scalp Stimulator for Dandruff
APPLY ONE TO THREE TIMES A WEEK

1 tablespoon cayenne pepper

1 cup oil (olive, sesame, sunflower, or almond)

Warm the oil on the stove or in the microwave, and mix in the cayenne pepper.

Massage well into the scalp for 10 minutes. Leave on overnight.

As I explained, the Nighttime Scalp Stimulator is a *nightly* treatment, while the Super Scalp Stimulator is a *weekly* treatment. *Do them both.*

The Super Scalp Stimulator is exactly what the name implies: a powerful scalp stimulator. It is to be used once a week in conjunction with the three other special treatments: the Slougher Cocktail, the Mud Pack, and the Protein Pack.

This once-a-week stimulation treatment is not a replacement for the nightly applications of the Nighttime Scalp Stimulator.

Super Scalp Stimulator
APPLY ONCE A WEEK

2 teaspoons Nighttime Scalp Stimulator

2 teaspoons basil oil (if available, otherwise use

2 teaspoons rosemary oil)

1 teaspoon white iodine

½ teaspoon castor oil

Put ingredients in an amber glass bottle with a glass dropper top. Close tightly and shake well to mix. Label.

Apply Super Scalp Stimulator to the scalp in the same way you do the Nighttime Scalp Stimulator. Massage for 10 minutes, then leave on 10 minutes longer.

Do not rinse.

Continue with the next step—the Slougher Cocktail (see page 51).

Step Four: Slough it Off

I introduced my Slougher Cocktail to the public on national television—on *The Merv Griffin Show*, to be exact—when I applied it to the famous bald head of Don Rickles. I have demonstrated it on *Late Night with David Letterman* as well as other shows, and no matter how many times I have shown it on TV or talked about it in interviews, the public response has been overwhelming. People love it!

Sloughing is the most effective way to dissolve wax buildup and remove dead cells caused by improper washing and insufficient rinsing, as well as not brushing properly. These impurities, as well as dust and pollution, clog the pores of the scalp and smother the root before the hair has a chance to grow.

Applied to the scalp with a soft toothbrush, the Slougher Cocktail loosens scaling such as dandruff and seborrhea while stimulating blood circulation through the scalp.

Be sure to use every ingredient in the Slougher Cocktail recipe because each one has a specific purpose, and together they work to totally cleanse your scalp.

Slougher Cocktail

APPLY ONCE A WEEK

¼ cup vodka

10 aspirin tablets

2 Alka-Seltzer tablets

2 teaspoons Scalp Shampoo (see page 57)

1 teaspoon cayenne pepper

In a small glass bowl, gently stir all the ingredients together until the tablets are dissolved.

Section your hair from the hairline, a little at a time. Using a soft toothbrush, apply the Slougher to your scalp and rub in a gentle, circular motion until your entire head is covered with Slougher. *Do not scrub too hard, you are not scouring a pot!*

Once you have covered your scalp, massage the remaining Slougher into the ends of your hair. This will dissolve any oily residue there.

An alternative slougher for oily hair uses white willow bark.

Willow Bark Alternative Slougher Cocktail for Oily Hair

2 tablespoons dried white willow bark

1 cup witch hazel

16 ounces pure water

Place the dried white willow bark in 16 ounces of water and bring to a boil. Turn off heat, steep for 1 hour. Let it cool down, then strain and pour into a glass bottle.

Put 1 cup of witch hazel in a spray bottle and add 1 tablespoon of the White Willow Bark formula. Add a drop of rosemary or lavender oil to make it smell good (this is optional). Spray on the roots of the hair to dissolve wax buildup.

If your scalp gets oily during the day, you can spray this formula on the roots anytime to freshen the hair.

Apply the next treatment without rinsing this one.

Step Five: Control Excess Oils

Beauty-conscious women have known about the value of mud and clay in caring for the skin and hair since the days of Cleopatra, at least. Now I am going to share this secret with all of you!

When I speak of mud, I am not talking about the mud that children track in from the backyard, but a mixture of fuller's earth and neutral henna.

Fuller's earth is a highly absorbent substance made of very pure clay and a natural, sandlike powder. Its gentle, absorbent quality is the very reason I use it.

The other ingredient in this very special recipe is neutral henna. This famous Egyptian herbal compound has been used in cosmetics and medicines for thousands and thousands of years. It makes an excellent hair wash, rinse, or dye, depending upon the strength of the solution you use. The powdered leaves can be mixed with other herbs to make different-colored natural semipermanent dyes.

For our purposes, we will be using neutral (color-free) henna. It leaves no color in the hair shaft but does wonderful things to the body of your hair.

Both fuller's earth and neutral henna absorb the oils from the scalp and act as healing agents for an irritated scalp.

Mud Pack

APPLY ONCE A WEEK

1 cup fuller's earth

1 cup neutral henna

Combine fuller's earth and neutral henna in a plastic bag with a zipper top or in a glass jar with a tight-fitting lid. Shake powders together to mix thoroughly. In a glass bowl, combine 2 tablespoons Mud Pack powder with 2-3 tablespoons boiling water. Add enough water to make a smooth, thick paste the consistency of oatmeal.

Using a pastry brush, apply the Mud Pack to your head. Work into your scalp and then rub into the ends of your hair. Do not worry about massaging the mud into your scalp because it is too thick. Leave on for 30 minutes.

Rinse thoroughly with warm or cool water.

Step Six: The Right Way to Shampoo

Shampooing removes the grime and dirt that builds up in your hair follicles as you move about through your day. For the papilla to

function properly, that grime and dirt needs to be removed—*daily.*
Additionally, your skin is constantly producing fresh skin cells,
pushing the older, dead cells to the surface. Shampooing removes
those dead cells from the scalp, allowing the skin to "breathe" properly. In short, you must shampoo each and every day.

This is particularly important for people who are suffering
from hair loss. Many people with this condition irrationally
believe that shampooing aggravates the condition by accelerating
the rate of alopecia, and choose to simply rinse their hair with
plain water. This couldn't be further from the truth. Just water-
ing the scalp allows the level of sebum trapped in the follicles to
build up. Moreover, that sebum also traps the grime and dirt collected from everyday life, eventually choking off the follicles and
worsening the condition.

*Set aside your fears. You must shampoo (or dry shampoo)
every day. Period.*

When shampooing, remember to use your fingertips to massage the scalp and disperse the lather through the hair. Do not
use the palms of the hands, as this could easily be too harsh and
may cause breakage of the hair shafts, resulting in eventual hair
loss. A gentle massage is an excellent way to invigorate the scalp,
which increases blood flow to the papilla and stimulates hair
growth (more about massage later). Rinse with cool or lukewarm
water.

The formulas included here are very gentle, and don't work
like the commercial shampoos you wisely disposed of. First of
all, they may appear thinner than you're used to, and they don't
leave your hair squeaky-clean. That "squeaky-clean" feeling was

actually a result of those commercial shampoos stripping away every last ounce of protective oil from under the cuticles of the hair shafts, which does not promote the health of the hair shafts. These recipes will clean your hair of the excess oil and dirt, while conditioning your hair to feel soft.

Until now, probably no one has ever told you to wash your hair every day with two different shampoos, but that is what I'm pre-scribing. One shampoo is for your scalp, and the other is for your hair.

This is because your hair and your scalp are entirely different, with entirely different requirements for a cleansing product. Each cleanser has a specific purpose. Used in conjunction, they clean both hair and scalp to perfection.

The Scalp Shampoo supports the Slougher in keeping the scalp clean. Daily cleansing with this shampoo, along with the weekly Slougher treatments, will eliminate any impurities that stick to the scalp, such as dust and dirt, as well as oil, which, if it is left on the scalp, will clog the pores. It also has an astringent, antiseptic effect on the scalp, balancing it and bringing it to a nor-mal state.

The Hair Shampoo removes impurities and dirt from the hair shaft itself, gently cleansing and adding body to the hair without any drying effect.

Use the Scalp Shampoo first, rinse with tepid water, then use the Hair Shampoo, and rinse again with tepid water. You'll then finish with the Protective Sealing Lotion, and if you need a styling aid, use the Volume Enhancing Styling Formula. Both of these are described in upcoming chapters.

This shampooing technique should be used daily. If you work out or swim during the day and wash your hair a second time, use only the Hair Shampoo for the second washing.

If you run into a time crunch and really can't shampoo one day, I've included a Dry Shampoo formula.

The key ingredient in these shampoos is castile soap, in liquid or lotion form. Castile is a fine, hard, unscented soap, usually white or cream-colored, named for the region of Spain where it was first made. All soaps are essentially made of either animal or vegetable fat combined with an alkali, such as sodium hydroxide or potassium hydroxide. This combination engenders a chemical reaction called *saponification*: the process by which fat is turned into soap. Pure castile soap is usually made with excellent quality oils and fats and a minimal amount of alkalis. If you can, avoid castile soaps with additives. These can work against the positive effects of the herbs you'll be adding yourself, causing more damage.

If you are unable to find liquid or lotion castile soap, you can easily make your own by shaving a bar of pure castile soap, preferably made with olive oil and no additives, into a quart of hot water. Let it simmer over low heat until all the soap chips have dissolved, or cover and let it sit overnight until they have dissolved. This viscous lotion is the basis for both the Scalp Shampoo and the Hair Shampoo. If you are unable to purchase pure castile soap in any of its commercially prepared forms—liquid, powder, or bar—you can use a soapwort formula. Soapwort is an herb that has natural lathering and cleansing properties.

Soapwort (Alternative to Castile Soap)

16 ounces pure water

4 tablespoons soapwort stems and leaves

Put the soapwort in a saucepan and pour enough water over it to completely cover the stems and leaves. Let it steep in the cold water for 4 hours, then bring to a boil and simmer for 10 minutes. Allow to cool, then strain. Discard the herbs and use the liquid in the following shampoo recipes.

You will prepare the herbs used in each of these shampoos by making an infusion (or tea) for each, and straining the liquid into 1/2 cup of liquid castile soap or soapwort formula.

Scalp Shampoo

APPLY ONCE A DAY

1 heaping tablespoon crushed basil leaves

1 heaping tablespoon lavender flowers

1 heaping tablespoon rosemary leaves

3 cups boiling water

½ cup liquid castile soap

Make an infusion of the herbs by boiling them in the water for at least 10 minutes (longer if possible). Strain, then discard the leaves. Allow the water to cool, then add it to the castile soap. Store in a nonbreakable bottle. Label.

Use 1 teaspoon Scalp Shampoo per washing. Apply to wet hair. Massage into scalp, adding a little water at a time to work into a lather.

Rinse thoroughly, using tepid water. Then wash with Hair Shampoo.

Hair Shampoo

APPLY ONCE A DAY

1 heaping tablespoon nettles

1 heaping tablespoon crushed sage

1 heaping tablespoon chamomile flowers

3 cups boiling water

½ cup liquid castile soap

Make an infusion of the herbs by boiling them in the water for at least 10 minutes (longer if possible). Strain, then discard the leaves. Allow the water to cool, then add it to the castile soap. Store in a nonbreakable bottle. Label.

Use only 1 teaspoon of this highly concentrated shampoo per washing, massaging it gently into your hair. Rinse thoroughly with Tea Rinse (see page 60).

After using these very special shampoo products, you will not want to go back to the products sold in the store. I've had clients tell me that their old brands of shampoo made their hair feel gummy and sticky after they had been using these highly concentrated scalp and hair cleansers. They leave no residue on your hair, so you won't need to change shampoos every few months.

Make enough of your private-label scalp and hair shampoos to have in your gym bag so you can use them after working out, and for your travel bag so you'll have them with you while you're on the road.

If you must miss a shampoo, use this Dry Shampoo formula:

Dry Shampoo
2 ounces powdered orrisroot

2 ounces arrowroot powder

1 drop of peppermint oil

Mix together in a glass bottle and shake well.

Separate hair into small sections, and apply to scalp with a soft toothbrush. Brush hair for 5 minutes to remove powder, then style (don't forget to wash your hairbrush, even after the dry shampoo).

Step Seven: Strengthen the Hair Shaft

The grand finale to the daily treatment regimen is a Protective Sealing Lotion that will flatten the hair's cuticle and restore the 2 percent acid mantle to the hair and scalp.

This is a delicate balance that is easily disturbed, especially if there is any soapy residue left in the hair and on the scalp after washing. The result of this simple treatment will be hair that is squeaky clean and absolutely shimmering with life.

Wash your hair according to the instructions in Step Four, and rinse it until the water runs clear after your second lathering with the Hair Shampoo (or your alternative shampoo). As a final rinse, pour a diluted solution of Protective Sealing Lotion and warm water through your hair.

Once again, you are working with a highly concentrated product, so a little goes a long way. The following recipe makes enough to last for more than two weeks.

Protective Sealing Lotion

APPLY ONCE A DAY

32-ounce bottle apple cider vinegar

1 heaping tablespoon dried rosemary

1 heaping tablespoon dried sage

1 heaping tablespoon nettles

1 heaping tablespoon dried basil

1 heaping tablespoon chamomile flowers

Crush herbs gently with a mortar and pestle, or rub them between the palms of your hands to break them up a little.

Heat the apple cider vinegar in an enamel or glass pot. Add the herbs. Cover and simmer over low heat for 30 minutes.

Cool, then strain and funnel the liquid back into the vinegar bottle for safekeeping. Label and store in the refrigerator. (Don't forget to label your Protective Sealing Lotion. Nothing in it would harm you, but I don't think this souped-up vinegar would be very tasty in a salad dressing).

Mix ¼ cup Protective Sealing Lotion with 1 quart tepid water. Pour through your hair; rinse with the Tea Rinse.

Tea Rinse

1 tablespoon nettles

1 tablespoon dried horsetail

1 tablespoon dried rosemary

1 tablespoon dried sage

1 tablespoon dried basil

1 tablespoon dried Indian hemp

1 tablespoon dried chaparral

½ gallon water

Boil the water. Turn off the heat and steep the herbs in the boiling water until it makes a strong tea. Strain and store the tea in a glass bottle. Label.

Pour a cup of Tea Rinse through your hair. If you'd like, you can hold a bowl under your head to catch the Tea Rinse and then pour it through your hair again.

Briskly rub your hair and scalp with terry cloth towels, or better yet, "mitts" made of terry cloth. This will not only absorb much of the excess water but will also stimulate circulation in your scalp.

Comb your hair with your fresh, clean comb and then style.

To increase your hair's body and provide added protection to new growth when drying either hair or scalp, use the Volume Enhancing Styling Formula in Chapter Nine.

7

Shampoo Alternatives:

Special Herbs for Your Unique Hair

Many things can be accomplished in the shampoo step in addition to thoroughly cleaning the hair and scalp. You can enhance the color of your hair, you can adjust for an oily or dry scalp, strengthen the hair shaft, or you can treat dandruff. Because these things can be incorporated into your shampoo, in this chapter I am offering a chart listing many readily available herbs that can be infused and added to the Essential Shampoo Formula below to adjust for all hair types and colors for each member of your family. You would simply use the Essential Shampoo Formula in place of the Hair Shampoo in Step Four.

Essential Shampoo Formula

16 ounces pure water

Herb(s) of your choice

1 bar pure castile soap

From the chart of herbs below, select the herbs for your particular hair type. Make an infusion by combining 1 teaspoon of each of the herbs of your choice in 8 ounces of boiling water. Turn off the stove and let the herbs steep for about 6 hours. Strain and discard the herbs, then gently reheat water.

Now, bring another 8 ounces of pure water to a rolling boil in a second pot. Shave the bar of pure castile soap with a knife or grater. Stir the soap shavings into the boiling water until fully melted.

Add 2 tablespoons of the melted castile soap to the warm herbal infusion, constantly stirring until well mixed. Dilute with additional pure water, as needed. Remove from heat and cool. Pour into a small jar or squeeze bottle. Give it a good shake before each use.

The remaining melted castile soap can be stored and saved for use as needed.

The following chart lists several useful herbs that can be infused and combined with the Essential Formula. The chart notes their common properties, and the general hair types for which they are most effective. You can select several combinations of herbs and experiment to your own particular needs and taste. It is recommended that you make more than one shampoo so that you can alternate according to your hair type. For those with oily hair, you should rotate every other day with a shampoo specific for normal hair; otherwise, your hair will be stripped of all oils, becoming dry and brittle. For those with dry hair, you should alternate with a normal solution every other day as well. This will prevent your hair from becoming too oily, which will clog the follicles and lead to unwanted damage. People with normal hair should alternate between a normal solution, an oily solution, and a dry solution. This will help to keep your pH levels balanced.

Herbs and Their Properties	Normal	Dry Hair	Oily Hair
Burdock: Stimulates circulation of the scalp.	X	X	X
Chamomile: Anti-inflammatory properties; heals scalp irritations; a natural hair tonic that also has a lightening effect, producing yellow highlights.	X	X	
Chaparral: Stimulates circulation of the scalp.	X	X	X
Comfrey: The leaves can heal irritated scalp conditions when used in an infusion.		X	
Elderflower: Anti-inflammatory properties; heals scalp irritations; gentle hair stimulant.	X	X	
Eucalyptus: Anti-inflammatory properties; heals scalp irritations; assists in regulating sebum production; and is a deep-cleaning agent.			X
Garlic: Stimulates circulation of the scalp and promotes hair growth; heals scalp irritations; controls flaking; and heals eczema.	X	X	X
Horsetail: Stimulates circulation of the scalp; also a good source of silica, which promotes strength of hair shaft.	X	X	X
Indian hemp: Stimulates circulation of the scalp.	X	X	X
Lavender: Gentle hair stimulant; regulates pH levels; promotes body and shine of hair shaft; leaves a pleasant, soothing scent.	X		X
Lemon balm: Gentle cleansing herb that removes excess oil and sebum.			X

Herbs and Their Properties	Normal	Dry Hair	Oily Hair
Lemongrass: Gentle cleansing herb that removes excess oil and sebum.			X
Lemon verbena: Cleanser and scalp stimulant.			X
Licorice: Contains a compound that prevents testosterone from being converted to DHT in men.	X	X	X
Marshmallow root: Has a potent conditioning and softening effect.		X	
Nettle (aka stinging nettle): Stimulates circulation of the scalp, and is a cleanser.	X	X	X
Parsley: Promotes the health of the sebaceous glands; heals scalp irritations; conditions and stimulates the hair.	X	X	X
Peppermint: Stimulates circulation of the scalp; acts as a gentle antiseptic.	X		X
Red Clover: Gentle cleansing herb.		X	
Rosemary: Controls flaking and heals eczema; great for dark hair; also stimulates circulation of the scalp.	X	X	X
Sage: Helps reduce the level of sebum production in the sebaceous glands; stimulates circulation of the scalp.			X
Thyme: Cleansing and tonic properties; leaves a terrific scent.	X		X
Yarrow root: Helps reduce the level of sebum production in the sebaceous glands.			X

You can try several combinations of these herbs: lavender and rosemary with chamomile gives a nice herbal scent. Chamomile and marshmallow root are great for light hair; while sage, comfrey, and rosemary are excellent for darker hair. The following chart lists several useful herbs that can be infused and combined with the shampoo formulas in this chapter for particular hair colors:

Black hair	Black henna, black malva, indigo, lavender; red henna or cloves can be added for reddish highlights
Blond or light hair	Acacia flowers, black cherry bark, broom, calamus, chamomile, marigold, marshmallow root, orange flower, orrisroot, quassia chips, saffron, St. John's wort, turmeric, yellow mullein flowers
Blue/White hair	Bachelor's button, blue malva, comfrey root, lavender (not to be used on dry hair), white chamomile flowers
Brown hair	Aloe leaf, cassia bark, cloves, maidenhair, yarrow root
Brunette hair	Cloves, comfrey leaf, jaborandi, lavender (not to be used on dry hair), marjoram, mint, quassia chips, raspberry, rosemary, sage, sassafras; also herbs listed for brown or black hair
Gray/dingy hair	Hollyhock (turns dingy gray hair silver with bluish highlights)
Red hair	Cloves, cochineal, marigold, red henna, red hibiscus, witch hazel bark

Aloe Vera and Jojoba

While not technically classified as herbs, aloe vera and jojoba can also be beneficial adjuncts to your shampoo formula. Stabilized aloe vera purchased in either a powder, gel, or concentrate works to strengthen the outer cuticle of the hair shafts, giving them a uniform, more reflective appearance—in short, promoting tangle-free, shiny hair. The antiseptic properties of aloe vera also work to heal the scalp and relieve it of eczema and flaking. Jojoba oil has long been acknowledged as a cure for many hair ailments, ranging from alopecia to eczema. Structurally, it is very similar to the sebum in your hair. This gives it the ability to attract and draw out unwanted sebum embedded in the follicles. Additionally, it tends to soothe the scalp, progressively decreasing excess sebaceous gland secretions, and heals irritations and the flaking of the scalp.

Strengthening Formula

Willow leaves have been noted to strengthen hair and stimulate an accelerated rate of growth. Here's another shampoo formula that also includes birch leaves, which are renowned for their unique ability to fortify the hair structure.

Willow and Birch Strengthening Shampoo Formula

6 cups pure water

1 cup willow leaves

1 cup birch leaves

6 tablespoons pure castile soap shavings

Bring the water to a boil, then add the willow and birch leaves. Cover and reduce heat, then steep for no less than 2 hours. Remove from heat and let stand until cool. Strain and discard the leaves.

Gently reheat the infused water, and then add the pure castile soap shavings, constantly stirring until melted. Remove from heat and cool. Pour into a small jar or squeeze bottle. Let the mixture stand at least 24 hours before first use. Always give it a vigorous shake before use.

To receive the maximum benefits of this strengthening formula, gently massage into your scalp and leave it in for 10 minutes. Rinse thoroughly with cool or tepid water.

Comfrey root, nettles, peppermint, or quassia chips can be infused along with this formula to heal dry itchy scalp and eczema.

Raw Egg

Raw egg, which is mostly protein, can give hair (which is 97 percent protein) a boost with extra body and shine. Beat 1 raw egg, then combine with 1 tablespoon of either the Essential Shampoo or Willow and Birch Strengthening Shampoo Formulas. Shampoo as you would normally, but make sure you rinse your hair for at least 1 minute with cool or cold water. Warm water will poach the egg, leaving quite a mess in your hair. Since raw egg spoils quickly, it is recommended that you don't make this too far in advance. Be sure to refrigerate it, if you aren't going to use it immediately.

Beer

Since the Egyptians invented it over 4,000 years ago, beer has been recognized to have the ability to give hair more bounce, body, and shine. Beer can also be added to either the Essential or Willow and Birch Formulas. Heat 1 cup of your favorite beer (keep it to a light lager, like Rolling Rock or Budweiser) in a saucepan. Bring it to a slow boil until the liquid is reduced to ½ cup. Let it cool, then stir in 1 cup of the shampoo of your choice. Store in a jar or squeeze bottle. Shampoo as you normally would.

Other Shampoo Alternatives: Damaged Hair, Oily Scalp, Dandruff

Pre-Shampoo for Dry or Damaged Hair

FOR CHEMICALLY DAMAGED HAIR, APPLY IN THE MORNING

1 teaspoon honey

2 teaspoons olive oil

1 egg yolk

Combine honey and olive oil until blended, adding beaten egg yolk in slowly.

With pastry brush, apply to hair in small strands. Wrap your hair in a hot towel (or a shower cap will do), leave in for 15 minutes, then shampoo in cool water, then warm.

LemonAid Shampoo for Oily Scalp

3 tablespoons vodka

1 tablespoon lemon juice

2 ounces castile soap

1 quart distilled water

Grate soap into 1 quart distilled boiling water, then lower heat until soap dissolves. In a blender, whip the mixture, then beat in the alcohol and lemon juice. Cool, then shampoo. Store leftover shampoo in a labeled container.

Aromatic Dandruff Shampoo

8 ounces Hair Shampoo (see page 58)

8 drops rose geranium oil

8 drops lemon oil

8 drops rosemary oil

Add oils into shampoo, shake well, and apply.

8

Special Treatments:

Cream Rinses and Conditioners

S hampoos are intended to cleanse by removing unwanted particles and oils. Conditioners are designed to restore the proteins and moisture to the hair cuticles, follicles, and scalp. However, most conditioners available on the market are really just cream rinses intended to soften the hair, containing synthetic silicone derivatives, such as Dimethicone, to detangle the hair for combing and brushing. Other ingredients commonly used in commercial conditioners include propylene glycol, isopropyl alcohol, formaldehyde, FD&C Red Dye #4, synthetic fragrance, mineral oil, petrolatum, and tallow, all of which build up in the hair shafts and lead to damage. There are plenty of natural products sold in many commercial conditioners, such as ginseng, aloe, green tea, plants, fruits, and flowers, but the quantities are insufficient to have any effect beyond enhancing the product's fragrance.

If you feel that your hair care program should include a conditioner, either because your hair is dry or damaged or tends to tangle, here is an Essential Conditioning Formula that can be used as a cream rinse three to four times a week, after shampooing.

Essential Conditioning Formula

8 ounces pure water

1 teaspoon herb(s) of your choice (see pages 65–66)

1 scoop powdered soy or whey protein

Begin by making an herbal infusion from the herbs. Bring the water to a boil, and then add 1 teaspoon of each of the herbs of your choice. Turn off the stove, and let the herbs steep for about 6 hours. Strain and discard the remains of the herbs. Add protein powder, stirring until well mixed. Store in a plastic squeeze bottle, and label.

Use only after shampooing by massaging onto the hair with your fingertips. If you have oily hair, apply to the ends of the hair only, avoiding the roots; administering it to your scalp will inadvertently increase the production of oil in the follicles. Let stand for 3 minutes, then rinse with cool or tepid water. Proceed with a rinse, described in the second half of this chapter.

As with the shampoo formulas, the Essential Conditioning Formula is also a good opportunity to use herbs that enhance hair color through herbal infusion. Look on page 67 for a guide.

Once-a-Week Herbal Oil Treatment

This once-a-week herbal oil treatment can be quite potent for restoring damaged hair with split ends.

Herbal Oil Treatment Formula

1 cup olive oil

1 cup peanut oil

4 ounces herb(s) of your choice (see previous charts)

½ ounce rosemary or pure basil oil

Combine the olive and peanut oils with the herbs in a non-metal pot. Bring to a simmer, and continue heating until herbs are crisp. Strain the herbs, then pour 6 ounces of the infused oil into another bowl. Mix in the rosemary or basil oil. Store in a plastic squeeze bottle, and label.

Apply to the hair shafts, taking care to avoid the scalp and roots. Wrap your head in a warm towel, and then cover with a shower cap. Let stand for 1 hour. Rinse completely, then shampoo. (This formula can also be used as a scalp pack, and is especially good for healing a dry, inflamed scalp. The condition can be cleared up by applying this formula about three to four times a week *to the scalp only.* Thereafter, it can be used as a scalp pack once a week.)

Flour and Water Conditioner

Another hair-pack conditioner, which is often used in the best salons in Europe, is made from a simple mixture of flour and water. Rinsing it out may be a bit of work, but the results are worth the effort.

Flour Conditioning Formula

1 cup flour

1 cup water

Combine the flour and water into a paste.

Apply to dry hair and let stand for 15 to 20 minutes. Rinse thoroughly with cool water—hot water will make the paste hard to rinse out. Rinsing will probably take 5 to 10 minutes, but you will see that your hair is much more manageable and shiny. You can shampoo and rinse after using this formula.

Conditioner for Dry Hair
Molasses, which is the basis for rum, does wonders for dry hair.

Rum Conditioning Formula for Dry Hair
3 tablespoons rum

1 egg yolk

Combine the egg yolk and rum, mixing well.

After shampooing, pour the formula into your hair. Allow 10 minutes for absorption. Rinse with water as cool as you can stand. Warm or hot water will poach the egg, making quite a mess.

You can really simplify this formula by applying a half-cup of blackstrap molasses to your hair and allowing it to absorb for 20 minutes. Rinse with cool or tepid water. Blackstrap molasses can be drunk as a mineral supplement because it is rich in calcium, iron, niacin, phosphorus, potassium, riboflavin, and sodium—all of which are great for promoting the health of your scalp. One caveat, though: if you choose to drink it straight from the bottle, be sure to brush your teeth immediately after, since molasses is also known for its striking ability to promote tooth decay.

The following alternative cream rinse formula is excellent for dry and easily damaged hair, and should be used no more than once or twice a week. It is perishable and should be used immediately, yielding just enough for a single treatment.

Honey and Lemon Conditioning Formula

1 teaspoon almond oil

1 teaspoon avocado oil

1 teaspoon olive oil

1 egg yolk

1 tablespoon honey

1 tablespoon fresh lemon juice

Combine all of the ingredients and stir thoroughly. Use immediately.

After shampooing, massage the Honey and Lemon Formula into your hair and let stand for 5 to 10 minutes. Rinse.

Here's another one that is good for thin, dry, and easily damaged hair suffering from split ends. The mixture of gelatin and egg makes an excellent protein and lecithin cream rinse formula for weekly use.

Gelatin and Egg Formula

1 tablespoon unflavored gelatin

¼ cup water

1 egg yolk

2 tablespoons fresh lemon juice

Gently warm the water, then stir in the gelatin until dissolved.

Allow to cool, then add the egg yolk and lemon juice, stirring until well mixed.

After shampooing, massage the Gelatin and Egg Formula into your hair and let stand for 2 to 3 minutes. Rinse with cool water.

Conditioner for Oily Hair

For oily hair, cantaloupe works well as a conditioner.

Cantaloupe Conditioning Formula for Oily Hair

½ cup fresh cantaloupe

Mash the melon with a fork until smooth.

Massage the cantaloupe into your scalp and leave on your hair for at least 10 minutes. Rinse with cool water. (As a further recommendation, you can eat the leftover cantaloupe.)

If your hair is long or dry, or if you have split ends despite frequent haircuts, you can use this Split End Hair Treatment daily. The nongreasy oils in this formula will be absorbed into the hair shaft and will keep the hair smooth, shiny, and healthy.

Split End Hair Treatment

1 teaspoon lavender oil

1 teaspoon basil oil

1 teaspoon rosemary oil

1 teaspoon nettle oil

Combine all oils together in a small dark bottle with an eyedropper and shake well.

Put a few drops on the palm of your hand and rub through your hair, then brush. The oils may be used all together, or you can combine only one or two.

9

Styling the Hair:

Natural Formulas to Replace Styling Gels and Mousses

Styling aids—from mousses to gels and blow dryers to styling wands—are as common as ice cream nowadays. Everyone uses them! We have our hair styled rather than just cut or barbered. We apply colors or rinses, perms or straighteners, anything we feel might make us more attractive.

Anyone who has hair and scalp problems, especially severe hair loss from either male pattern baldness or alopecia areata, will try just about anything on earth to make his or her hair look better or thicker or to restore lost hair while maintaining what hair is left.

Ironically, the latest additions to this growing trend in hair care and styling, especially mousses and gels, can be brutally damaging. In fact, they can be almost as harmful to both hair and scalp as that "greasy kid stuff" and oily tonic of the fifties and sixties or the alcohol-filled grooming aids that Grandpa might have used. Most of the popularly marketed products have alcohol in them. Others, although they may be alcohol-free, are full of chemicals that take their toll on the delicate composition of the hair.

Hairstyling lotions make the hair more pliable and keep it in place. This is accomplished by coating the hair shaft and soaking the layers of the cuticle. Strong chemicals, such as alcohol, can literally damage the interior structure of the hair if they are misused.

Once again, I turned to nature for a styling aid that cannot overdry or harm your hair, despite the fact that it adds body and bounce. Made of flaxseeds, it has a lot of holding power without any of the drying properties associated with chemically based products.

Volume Enhancing Styling Formula

APPLY ONCE A DAY

1 cup flaxseeds

3 cups water

Bring the water to a boil in a glass or enamel pot. Slowly stir the seeds into the boiling water and reduce heat. Simmer for 10 to 20 minutes, stirring constantly, until a gel-like lotion is formed.

Strain the lotion through a fine strainer or several layers of cheesecloth into a glass jar. Discard the seeds. Dilute with a little water if necessary to make it about the same consistency as the Scalp Shampoo. Label and store any remaining lotion in the refrigerator for up to six weeks. Take care that you don't put your fingers or comb into the solution, or you might contaminate it.

Pour a small amount into the palm of your hand. Rub it into your hair and comb to distribute the lotion, or pour a small quantity into a spray bottle and squirt a little bit into your hair, then comb to distribute the gel from the roots to the ends.

Volume Enhancing Styling Formula works just like the expensive hairstyling products, but it is perfectly safe for both hair and scalp and costs only pennies in comparison.

You will be amazed how light the Volume Enhancing Styling Formula feels on your hair, and best of all, how it doesn't become sticky when the air is humid. With the Volume Enhancing Styling Formula your hair will still feel clean at the end of the day.

Here are a few alternative styling formulas:

Egg Setting Formula

1 tablespoon egg white

4 tablespoons tepid water

Combine the water and egg whites with a whisk until the ingredients form a smooth lotion. If you are not intending on using this immediately, store in a small jar and refrigerate.

When washing your hair, remember to use cool water, or else the egg will poach on your scalp.

Sugar Spray Formula

1 tablespoon sugar

8 tablespoons warm water

Combine the sugar with the water, stirring until dissolved. Pour the formula in a spray bottle.

Apply to the hair either before or after styling. This is an old, tried-and-true formula that works very well. Since sugar does a good job of attracting bugs and bees, it's not recommended that you use this one during the spring and summer seasons.

Unflavored gelatin combined with water is another good essential styling gel from which there are several excellent variations you can try.

Essential Gelatin Styling Formula

1 cup water

1 teaspoon unflavored gelatin

Heat the water to just before the boiling point. Add the gelatin, stirring until completely dissolved. Remove from heat and allow to cool. The mixture is ready to use when firm to the touch. If you prefer the gel to be on the stiff side, cool in the refrigerator, although this mixture is just as effective when used at room temperature.

Use a small amount for styling either wet or dry hair.

Champagne is a combination of sugars and proteins, can be banded with the gelatin formula to thicken hair and add bounce.

Champagne Gelatin Styling Formula

½ cup water

½ cup champagne

1 tablespoon rosewater

1 teaspoon unflavored gelatin

Heat the water and dissolve the gelatin as in the Essential Gelatin Styling Formula. Add the champagne and rosewater and stir again. Pour in a wide jar, and place in the refrigerator to cool. When the formula has set, remove from the refrigerator. The mixture is ready to use when it reaches room temperature.

Almond oil added to the gelatin formula can restore hair that is damaged from the constant use of blow-dryers, curling irons, and rollers, while working as a very good styling gel.

Almond Oil Styling Formula

1-½ cups water

1 tablespoon unflavored gelatin

1 teaspoon glycerin

1 tablespoon almond oil

Heat the water and dissolve the gelatin as in the Essential Gelatin Styling Formula. Add the glycerin and almond oil, stirring until well blended. Remove from heat and pour into a wide glass jar. At this point the oil will probably rise to the top. Don't worry about it; just put the formula in the refrigerator and allow to cool for one hour. Stir the formula, recombining the oil and gelatin. Return to the refrigerator for one additional hour. Remove from the refrigerator. When the formula reaches room temperature, give it one more thorough stir, then it's ready to use.

This formula can be applied to either wet or dry hair to set and style.

The natural sugars in grapefruit work very well when combined with the proteins of the gelatin formula to hold the hair in place.

Grapefruit Styling Formula

½ cup water

1 tablespoon unflavored gelatin

½ cup fresh grapefruit juice

1 teaspoon glycerin

1 crushed vitamin C tablet

Heat the water and dissolve the gelatin as in the Essential

Gelatin Styling Formula. Add the remaining ingredients and stir until well mixed. Pour the mixture into a wide glass jar, and refrigerate until firm (about two hours). Remove from the refrigerator. When the formula reaches room temperature, give it one final stir. It's now ready for use on either dry or wet hair.

Tips for Safe Hairstyling

Don't brush hair when it's wet. If you do, the hair will break. Comb wet hair gently with a smooth-toothed comb. The teeth of the comb should have no rough, sharp edges.

Don't blow-dry your hair at the hottest temperature. Take a few more minutes and use a lower temperature. Even better, allow your hair to dry naturally whenever possible.

If you use rollers, set your hair on large ones without tension. Rolling the hair too tightly will put stress on the roots, causing breakage and loss. Use end papers if you use rollers.

Curling irons or electric rollers should be used at a low temperature. Hot curling tools can cause breakage and drying and can also overstimulate the sebaceous glands in the scalp. This means your scalp will be too oily!

Don't go out in the sun without protecting your hair with a hat. And never sunbathe without washing the salty sea water or chemical-filled pool water from your hair and then putting on a hat or scarf. Before swimming, rinse out any commercial styling gels, mousses, and sprays (which are full of alcohol and other chemicals) so these don't interact with the salt water or pool chemicals. Protect your hair and scalp by rubbing Nighttime Scalp Stimulator (page 48) into your scalp and the ends of your hair before going swimming or spending time in the sun.

In cold weather, protect your hair with a hat or scarf. Frigid temperatures can be as brutal on your hair as hot weather and pollution.

10

Natural Hair Colorants:

How to Color Your Hair Without Damaging It

Hair coloring has become as common today for men as for women. However, the chemicals used to strip or enhance the pigmentation in the cortex of the hair shaft are extremely harsh. After repeated use to maintain your color, these chemicals will inevitably lead to serious damage. No matter what your salon stylist may say, *it will fry your hair*. Particularly if you are experiencing hair loss or thinning, and you are serious about reversing your condition and restoring your scalp to its full health, *then you must immediately stop the use of chemical hair colorants*.

Fortunately, there are natural alternatives that do no damage to the hair, particularly if coloring is included as part of this program. You will need to do a sample test with many of the recipes (particularly those with henna) to make sure you have the right color. After mixing the recipes, select a small piece of hair from the nape of your neck—a place that is usually unnoticeable. Bind the selected hair tightly with a rubber band, then apply the mixture. Wrap your hair in plastic wrap, and then let stand for the recommended time in the recipe. Rinse the sample, and dry thoroughly. Check the color under a good strong light source, such as the sun. If you're satisfied with the tint, then proceed with the whole head.

Several of the recipes require more than one application, so they do not really require a test. Simply repeat the application until the desired color is achieved.

As listed in the chapters on shampoos, conditioners, and rinses, there are several herbs that, when used repeatedly over a period of days, can produce remarkable coloring results. Ingredients like chamomile flowers, rhubarb, and mullein can lighten the hair and give it a golden sheen. Sage, tea, and tobacco can be used to darken and mask gray hair. Hibiscus flowers are used to redden hair.

A basic rinse can be made with an infusion from the herbs listed on page 67:

Herbal Coloring Rinse
¼ cup herb(s) of your choice
2 cups pure water
Bring the water to a boil, then add the herb(s) of your choice. Reduce heat, cover and allow to simmer for 30 minutes. Remove from heat and cool. Strain into a jar or squeeze bottle. This can be used as a rinse after shampooing and conditioning.

Darkening and Covering Gray

Henna has been used for thousands of years to darken hair because it is a very good semipermanent dye that seals the cuticle layer of the hair shaft, locking in natural oils. This gives the hair enhanced shine and luster. While the color lasts as long as three to six months, it has the nice advantage of washing out gradually so you won't see the roots develop as your hair grows.

There is one caveat to using henna. Often, when initially applied, it leaves the hair looking brassy or dull. This is completely normal, as it requires an adjustment period of about three days before your cuticles will accommodate the color. After that, it should leave your hair looking quite shiny and lustrous.

Because henna comes in several different shades, it can be mixed to produce a wide variety of tints. For instance, red henna can be combined with brown to produce auburn. Once you've determined the desired shade (and after you've tested it), you're ready for the next step:

Henna Coloring Formula

½ cup pure henna powder (color mixture determined
*   from testing)*
¼ cup pure water (approximate)

Place the henna powder in a glass or ceramic bowl. Do not use a metal bowl or utensils, as the henna may chemically react to the metal. Plastic is not recommended either, since it may permanently stain the bowl.

Bring the water to a boil, and then slowly add to the henna while stirring. Add only enough water until you have the consistency of mud.

To apply, it is recommended that you use gloves to avoid staining your hands.

Apply the henna mixture to clean, dry hair, massaging well until the entire head is saturated to the ends of the hairs. Cover your head with a plastic shower cap.

To initiate the color absorption, you will need to warm your head. Sitting under a hair dryer, using a handheld blow dryer, or sitting in the sun are recommended. Continue for 15 to 45 minutes, depending upon how deep you want the color to be. The longer you leave it on, the darker the color will be.

Rinse your hair with warm water until the water is clear. Shampoo, then towel dry.

Indigo leaves can be added to the henna paste to make a deep black tint.

Indigo Henna Coloring Formula

¼ cup dark (or black) henna

22 heaping tablespoons indigo leaves, pounded

¼ cup pure water (approximate)

1 egg yolk

Corn oil

Combine the henna powder and indigo leaves in a glass or ceramic bowl. Bring the water to a boil, and then slowly add to the henna while stirring. Add only enough water until you have the consistency of mud.

Allow to cool, then stir in the egg yolk.

Massage the scalp and hair with corn oil to prevent drying, then apply the henna mixture, massaging well until the entire head is saturated to the ends of the hairs. Cover your head with a plastic shower cap.

Depending upon the desired shade of black in combination with your original hair color, it is recommended that you leave this on your hair for one to two hours.

Rinse thoroughly with cool water (you don't want scrambled egg in your hair), then shampoo and towel dry.

A coloring formula similar to the henna mixtures, which is applied to the scalp and allowed to dye the hair, can be derived from chamomile flowers.

Chamomile Coloring Formula

¼ cup chamomile flowers

2 cups pure water

8 tablespoons kaolin powder

1 egg yolk

Bring the water to a boil, then add the chamomile flowers. Reduce heat, cover, and allow to simmer for 30 minutes. Remove from heat and cool. Strain, and remove half of the liquid (which may be saved for an additional application). Stir in the kaolin powder and egg yolk.

Apply to the hair, cover with a plastic shower cap and leave in for 20 to 50 minutes. Rinse with cool water (warm water will cook the egg). This may be repeated until the desired shade is attained.

Sage, lavender, cinnamon, and tobacco are commonly used to darken hair and cover grays.

Darkening Rinse

¼ cup dried sage, or

¼ cup dried lavender, or

3 cinnamon sticks

2 cups pure water

Bring the water to a boil, and then add the sage, lavender, or cinnamon. Reduce heat, cover, and allow to simmer for 30 minutes. Remove from heat and cool. Strain into a jar or squeeze bottle. This can be used as a rinse after shampooing.

Sage Darkening Formula

¼ cup dried sage

2 teaspoons Lipton Tea (removed from the bags)

2 cups pure water

2 teaspoons rum

Bring the water to a boil, then add the sage and tea. Reduce heat, cover, and allow to simmer for 2 hours. Remove from heat and cool. Strain, then stir in the rum. Pour into a jar or squeeze bottle. Apply liberally to the hair, cover with a plastic shower cap, and leave in for 20 to 50 minutes. Rinse with cool water. This should be repeated five times a week to mask prematurely gray hair.

Lightening the Hair

Rhubarb can also be used to make a coloring formula.

Rhubarb Coloring Formula

¼ cup fresh rhubarb, finely chopped

2 cups pure water

8 tablespoons kaolin powder

1 egg yolk

½ teaspoon cider vinegar

1 teaspoon glycerin

Bring the water to a boil, then add the chopped rhubarb. Reduce heat, cover, and allow to simmer for 30 minutes. Remove from heat and cool. Strain, and remove half of the liquid (which may be saved for an additional application or as the basis for the Rhubarb Lightening Rinse). Stir in the kaolin powder, then the egg yolk, cider vinegar, and glycerin.

Apply to the hair, cover with a plastic shower cap, and leave in for 20 to 50 minutes. Rinse with cool water (warm water will cook the egg). This may be repeated to until the desired shade is attained.

This rhubarb rinse formula can be used to reinforce the highlights obtained from the Rhubarb Coloring Formula.

Rhubarb Lightening Rinse

¼ cup fresh rhubarb, chopped

2 cups pure water

Bring the water to a boil, then add the chopped rhubarb. Reduce heat, cover, and allow to simmer for 30 minutes. Remove from heat and cool. Strain into a jar or squeeze bottle. This can be used as a rinse after shampooing.

Highlights

Hibiscus flowers give a red highlight to light or dark brown hair.

Hibiscus Highlighting Rinse

Dried hibiscus flowers, or Hibiscus tea

Pure water

Bring the water to a boil, then add the flowers or tea. (The quantities will be determined by the amount of red highlighting that you desire.) Steep until the preferred shade appears in the water. Remove from heat and cool. Strain into a jar or squeeze bottle.

This can be used as a rinse after shampooing, and may require additional applications.

11

Massage Your Scalp:

Techniques that Make a Difference

Massage is almost as important to the success of my program as is the application of the treatments—and it feels so good!

Few people ever rub their heads unless they have a headache. It's such a pity, but what do you expect? Many people barely touch their loved ones every day. Why would I think they might consider cuddling themselves?

I feel so strongly about the benefits of massage for the scalp, neck, and face that I am going to teach you how to massage yourself and ask you to pass this technique along. You will absolutely glow, and so will your hair!

I want you to learn the proper techniques of scalp and neck massage—plus a few marvelous treats for your face—so that you can properly apply the treatments. Remember, I have asked you to *massage* the Stimulators into your scalp, and then to *massage* the Slougher Cocktail into your scalp...and *massage* is how you use the Scalp and Hair Shampoos!

Through my training in massage, I have learned techniques that actually increase the potency of the treatments. Scalp manipulation, as well as massage of the neck and face, stimulates blood

circulation through the scalp and neck, while relaxing and soothing the nerves in your head. Still another benefit of massage is
that it stimulates the muscles and activity of the various glands in
the scalp, especially the sebaceous glands. Stimulation, by the
way, doesn't mean they will be producing more oil as a result of
massage, but only that they will be working more efficiently.
Massage renders a tight scalp more flexible and helps maintain
the growth and health of the hair.

Learn to make these movements with a continuous, even
motion. Use the balls of your fingertips—never the nails—and
the cushions of your palms to stimulate all the activity in your
scalp, your neck, and even your face.

Never, ever jerk your neck about. Be gentle, not rough. Slide
your fingers through your hair and concentrate all your positive
energies on your scalp surface.

I asked my friend and client Ron Ronan about the benefits of
massage. He should know—he's a licensed massage therapist
who uses a variety of techniques to treat physical problems.
Ron has seen tense, pained patients relax almost immediately
after he has begun working on their heads and necks. "I think
there is something neurological in the benefits of scalp massage," he says. There are a lot of neurons (nerve centers) there.
As soon as you start to work on these, people immediately begin
to relax.

Ron tells me that he has had clients relax so completely on his
table while he was massaging their scalp, neck, and face that they
have actually gone to sleep. "There is something nurturing about
massage of the head and neck...I have had people tell me that

they have their hair shampooed and styled because they like the way if feels, even more than the way it looks."

Start your massage session with some simple facial exercises. They will get your circulation moving.

The Kiss: Pucker your lips together in an exaggerated kiss. Hold for a count of five; relax and repeat ten times.

Chewing: Open your mouth as wide as you can. Circle your jaws in a vast chewing motion. Move slowly and deliberately, chewing and chewing for a count of twelve.

The Lion: This famous yoga posture is also excellent for the face and scalp. Open your eyes as wide as you can, then open your mouth as wide as possible, and stick your tongue out as far as you can, pointing the tip downward, toward your chin. Hold for a count of fifteen; relax and repeat.

Scales: This super massage technique for the face that was created to ease the pain of Temporomandibular Joint Syndrome (TMJ). Place your fingertips on your cheeks, feeling that recess where your upper and lower teeth mesh as you chew or talk. Move your fingers as though playing scales on the piano, pressing as deeply and firmly as feels comfortable.

Neck Rolls: Complete your warm-ups by slowly rotating your head from side to side five times in each direction.

Hanging: Lie on your back on a bed or table. Hang your head off the edge so that blood circulation is increased through the neck and scalp. Breathe deeply and relax. Lie there for several minutes.

Next, try these simple scalp massage movements.

Forehead Manipulation: Hold your left hand across the back of your head to steady your neck. Relax your head into your hand. Place your right hand across your forehead, stretching your thumb and forefinger across your brow line. Move your hand slowly and firmly upward to one inch past your hairline. Repeat five times.

Scalp Manipulation: Place the palms of your hands firmly against your scalp above each ear. "Lift" the scalp in a circular movement, first with the hands at the side of your head, then with one hand at the top front and the other at the center back, right at the nape of your neck.

Sliding Movements: With your fingertips on either side of your head, slide your fingers firmly upward. Spread your fingertips until they meet on top of your head. Repeat five times.

Hairline Circles: Beginning at the hairline, place the fingers of both hands on the center of your hairline—right at your forehead. Massage around the hairline, concentrating on the areas of hair loss as you work your fingertips in a gentle circular motion. Work all the way around your hairline, including the temples, behind your ears, and across the back of your neck.

Crown Manipulations: Placing your fingertips at the crown, work in gentle circular movements throughout the crown. Work outward, moving forward to the temples and then back along the sides. Repeat five times.

Ear-to-ear Movements: Hold your left hand across your forehead, letting your head rest in the cup made by your palm. With the fingertips of your right hand, start behind your left ear and make gentle but steady circular motions along the base of your skull. If you are afraid of massaging too roughly, use the heel of your palm in a rotary movement from ear to ear. Repeat twice.

Zigzags: Using your fingertips only, work in a firm up and down motion, moving from side to side. Work from the crown to the neckline and then reverse the process, zigzagging from the nape to the crown. Repeat twice.

Pulling: Gently grasp small bunches of your hair firmly with your fingertips. Pull slowly—do not yank on your hair—for a count of three and release. Repeat, pulling small bunches of hair until your entire head of hair has been tugged.

Slant Board

In addition to your scalp massage, you can increase the circulation to your scalp by using a slant board. In addition, while you're on the slant board is the perfect time to massage your scalp.

The slant board originated in India and was initially known in the West as the Yoga Slant. You can purchase one in many department and health food stores. If you should find the price prohibitive, you can easily make a homemade slant board for a fraction of the price.

Lie on the slant board with your feet at the elevated end twice a day for a maximum of ten minutes at a time. The intention here is to use the earth's gravitational pull to force your blood to your scalp, increasing vasodilation and feeding the papilla in your follicles.

If you happen to own a back swing or gravity boots (recommended only for the very fit), these can be used instead of the slant board. If you have a condition of high blood pressure, you need to consult your physician, who will most likely advise you to stick to using the slant board.

Be sure to use caution when standing, as the increased level of blood suddenly draining from your head can cause dizziness.

12

Skincare and the Face:

Healthy Hair Comes With Healthy Skin

How you care for your face is a critical, and often disregarded, aspect in the overall health of your hair, and a determining factor in hair loss. This is particularly so for men, who are content to wash with a bar of soap and shave once a day, not really paying much attention at all to the condition of the epidermis on their face. Poor skincare promotes a buildup of sebum. This is the waxy oil that the sebaceous glands use to lubricate hair, and is the same oil that causes pimples and blackheads on the face.

A buildup of sebum on the face and forehead traps dead skin cells. Instead of falling away from the epidermis as they're supposed to do, they act to clog the pores. Up near the hairline, this discourages the proper functioning of the follicles and advances the conditions of damage and alopecia.

Regular hand and body soap should never be used to clean the face. The pH balance in these soaps strips away the necessary oils that are intended to lubricate a healthy face, and many of these soaps have antibacterial formulas that remove both the good and bad bacteria. Read the label on the soap: it ain't called *hand* or *body* soap for nothing.

A good facial routine has three basic steps applied both in the morning and evening: cleansing, toning, and moisturizing. Men should not worry: this won't take but a couple of additional minutes in the bathroom, and the results will be absolutely worth it. Not only will the well-being of your hair improve, but also the texture of your face will appear more vibrant and healthy.

Women are strongly urged not to skip over this part of the program. Most of you already have your favorite line of products you've relied on for years. Set them aside and try the formulas in this chapter. There are two particular advantages in using these recipes: first, they don't have any harsh chemicals (isopropyl alcohol and witch hazel, which are very drying and are no-nos) that can build up over time and damage your face. If you're using something from the drug store, you probably are doing more harm than good. If you're using a line of products from your favorite department store, then you're probably being gravely overcharged. The second advantage is that you won't be paying for any expensive advertising or licensing fees for the use of a famous designer's name on the label.

Cleansing

Using a cleanser will dislodge any dirt, grime, or oils collected in the pores. Oatmeal is a popular and exceptional natural cleanser. It's very mild and soothing, and is good for sensitive skin.

Oatmeal Facial Cleansing Formula
½ cup oatmeal

1 cup pure water

1 teaspoon glycerin

1-2 drops tincture of benzoin

Combine all ingredients in a food processor or blender. Puree into a creamy, smooth paste. Store in an airtight jar or plastic container. Label.

To use, apply a small amount to the face, gently scrubbing in circular motions over the cheeks, forehead, and nose. Make sure you reach all the way up to the hairline. Rinse well with warm water and pat dry.

A simpler formula can be made from combining three of the most effective cleansing grains.

3-Grain Facial Cleansing Formula

½ cup cornmeal

½ cup oatmeal

½ cup wheat germ

Stir the grains together, and then store in an airtight jar or plastic container.

To use, combine two teaspoons of the formula with just enough water to create a paste. Massage over your face, gently scrubbing in a circular motion. Rinse well with warm water and pat dry.

Toning

Using a toner will remove any remaining dirt and dead cells that may clog the pores, and they act as a humectant that prepares the skin for the third step, moisturizing. Toners should be applied with a white cotton ball or pure white facial tissue using a gentle circular motion on the skin. Be sure to apply it at the top of the forehead, just below the hairline.

Apple-Mint Facial Toning Formula

3 tablespoons fresh mint leaves

2 tablespoons apple cider vinegar

1 cup pure water

Finely chop the mint leaves. Combine with remaining ingredients in a jar. Screw on the lid and let stand for three days. Strain the formula through a layer of cheesecloth and discard the mint leaves. Store in a clean jar or squeeze bottle. Shake to mix well before each use.

Honey is particularly good for healing blemishes and softening the skin.

Honey Facial Toning Formula

1 tablespoon honey

1 teaspoon fresh lemon juice

1 tablespoon rosewater

2 tablespoons apple cider vinegar

Combine the ingredients in a jar or squeeze bottle. Shake until mixed before each use. To prevent the formula from feeling sticky, allow it to sit in the refrigerator for five days. If you don't want to wait that long, rinse your face with cool water after application.

Chamomile flowers are frequently used in cosmetics because they relieve inflammation and work to assist the skin in absorbing moisture.

Chamomile Facial Toning Formula

3 chamomile tea bags (100 percent chamomile only)
2 cups pure water
1-2 drops tincture of benzoin

Bring the water to a boil, and pour over the tea bags in a ceramic or glass heat-resistant bowl. Let steep for several hours until cool. Remove the tea bags, then stir in the tincture of benzoin. Store in a jar or squeeze bottle.

Moisturizing

The process of cleansing and toning is beneficial because you are removing the sebum and dirt that clog your pores (which can lead to hair loss and damage). It also strips away moisture, which is necessary to keep your skin healthy and vibrant. Keeping the skin moist is the crucial third step to subduing and balancing the oil production of the sebaceous glands.

Basic Facial Moisturizing Formula

¼ cup mineral oil
¼ cup stearic acid powder
½ teaspoon baking powder
2 tablespoons glycerin
1 cup pure water

Combine the mineral oil and stearic acid in a microwave-safe bowl.

Combine the remaining ingredients in a second microwave-safe bowl.

Heat the mineral oil and stearic acid in the microwave on High until the powder has melted and the mixture is clear, stirring occasionally.

Heat the water, baking powder, and glycerin in the microwave until it just starts boiling (about 2 minutes on High). Slowly stir the water into the oil solution. It will foam to twice its volume as carbon dioxide is released from the powder.

Pour the mixture into a blender and blend on High for 2 minutes, or until the mixture turns white and has a fluffy consistency. Spoon into a clean bowl and let stand until cool. Stir once again, then spoon into a jar for storage.

To use, massage a small amount onto your face and neck.

A modified version of this formula uses coconut oil, which is extremely nourishing for the skin.

Coconut Facial Moisturizing Formula

¼ cup coconut oil

¼ cup stearic acid powder

½ teaspoon baking powder

½ cup pure water

Combine the coconut oil and stearic acid in a microwave-safe bowl, and heat on High until melted.

Combine the baking powder and water in a second microwave-safe bowl. Stir until the powder is dissolved. Heat in the microwave until it just starts boiling (about 2 minutes on High). Slowly stir the water and baking powder into the oil solution. It will foam to twice its volume as carbon dioxide is released from the powder. Stir thoroughly. Let stand until cool. Stir once again, then spoon into a jar for storage.

To use, massage a small amount onto your face and neck.

Cornstarch can be used to make a formula that works wonders for severely dry or chapped skin.

Cornstarch Facial Moisturizing Formula

4 tablespoons cornstarch

4 tablespoons glycerin

4 tablespoons rose water

1 cup pure water

Combine all of the ingredients in a microwave-safe bowl and stir until thoroughly mixed. Heat on High (stirring every 30 seconds) until boiling and the mixture turns thick. Remove from the microwave and let stand until cool. Spoon into a jar for storage.

Should this jellylike formula thicken over time, just stir in one tablespoon of water at a time until the formula thins enough to use.

Honey can be used to make a very simple moisturizing formula.

Honey Facial Moisturizing Formula

2 tablespoons honey

24 drops almond oil

Combine the ingredients in a glass or ceramic bowl. Whip the oil and honey until they are completely mixed. Pour into a small jar, and store in the refrigerator.

To use, apply a tiny amount to each cheek and forehead. Massage gently, working in a circular motion up toward the hairline (make certain you don't get this in your hair). Use sparingly.

These three steps—cleansing, toning, and moisturizing—constitute a daily routine that will promote skin care and prevent hair loss and damage.

Now there is one more step to caring for your face that you will need to do once a week:

Facial Masks

A once-a-week mask will be very beneficial. It will help to unclog the pores of your face, remove dead cells and any remaining oil or other impurities, heal blemishes, and replace lost moisture while soothing the skin.

An added benefit to having a weekly mask is the fact that it requires you to relax, to remain calm and quiet for twenty to thirty minutes. Once a week, you are guaranteed to have half an hour to let everything go and pamper yourself. Having time to be alone, to meditate, or to simply reduce the stress in your life is an important factor in reversing hair loss and damage.

Once again, oatmeal makes a good cleanser, and because it is rich in protein and nutrients like magnesium, iron, potassium, and phosphate, it's nourishing for the skin. Select one of the following formulas for your skin type:

Oatmeal Mask Formula for Normal Skin

½ cup cooked oatmeal

1 tablespoon almond oil

1 egg

Oatmeal Mask Formula for Dry Skin

½ cup cooked oatmeal

½ banana, mashed

1 tablespoon honey

1 egg yolk

Oatmeal Mask Formula for Oily Skin

½ cup cooked oatmeal

½ cup apple, mashed

1 tablespoon fresh lemon juice

1 egg white

Combine all of the ingredients in a bowl and mix until a smooth paste is formed.

To use, apply to the face, and let stand for about 20 minutes. Rinse with tepid water. Pat dry, then apply a moisturizing formula derived from the aforementioned recipes.

Brewer's yeast is rich in vitamins, and is an excellent source for the proteins your skin requires. It comes in either a powder or in tablets, and can be found at most health food stores and many larger supermarkets.

Brewer's Yeast Mask Formula

1 teaspoon powdered brewer's yeast, or 6 tablets of brewer's yeast, crushed

1 tablespoon buttermilk or plain yogurt

Combine the ingredients in a bowl and mix together until smooth. Store in the refrigerator.

Apply evenly to the face, and leave until dry, about 20 minutes. Rinse with tepid water. Pat dry, then apply a moisturizing formula derived from the aforementioned recipes.

Clay does a terrific job of drawing out trace impurities and sebum, while refining the texture of your skin. The following is a classic formula that has been used for centuries.

Clay Mask Formula

1 tablespoon clay powder

2-3 tablespoons pure water

Mix together the clay and water in a ceramic bowl, adding only one teaspoon of water at a time until a smooth paste forms.

Apply the formula to your face, covering all areas except the eyes. Allow the clay to dry for about 20 to 30 minutes. Rinse with warm water. When the mask has been removed, rinse with cool water to close the pores. Pat dry, then apply a moisturizing formula derived from the aforementioned recipes.

13

You Are What You Eat:

How Nutrition—Vitamins, Minerals, and Herbs— Improves the Health of Your Hair

Just like the nails on your toes and fingers and the skin cells on the outermost layer of your epidermis, the hair you see on your scalp is fundamentally dead tissue. However, the follicle structure imbedded in the second and third layers of the epidermis is very much alive and is intricately dependent on the circulation of the blood through the body. Without a proper balance of nutrients, minerals, proteins, essential fatty acids, and trace minerals, the papilla will not properly synthesize proteins into keratin and produce healthy hair cells. Accordingly, the resulting hair growth will be less than optimal.

Clinical studies have shown a strong connection between hair loss and deficiencies in the class of B-complex vitamins. While it may appear to be an issue that could not possibly affect Western cultures due to the overabundance of food available, nothing could be further from the truth. Whole grains such as rice and wheat, while organically rich in B-complex, are commonly processed before they reach the market shelf. Consequently, they are stripped of many of their vital nutrients. The prevailing practice in most

Western households of oversteaming vegetables removes many of the B vitamins since they are water-soluble. The emphasis on fast and processed foods in the modern diet often supplants the intake of raw leafy greens, another superior source of B vitamins. This is further complicated by the fact that our Western diet is heavy in white flour, sugar, and refined grains. So that our bodies can digest these refined carbohydrates, the Bs that we do manage to ingest often get redirected to supporting their assimilation rather than nourishing our bodies.

Nicotine, caffeine, grain alcohol, and sugar are common stimulants that work like a two-edged sword affecting hair loss and the vitality of your hair. As they move through your system, they devour nutrients that are missing from their chemical structures. They also overwork the adrenal glands, eventually depleting them and increasing the nutritional requirements of your body. Most significantly, this raises the androgen levels in the bloodstream. Androgens are the hormones that convert the enzyme 5-alpha reductase into DHT. DHT restricts vasodilation to the papilla, eventually leading to hair loss.

Animal products—such as milk, butter, fatty meats, and cheese—are very common in Western diets. These foods increase the levels of cholesterol, which is synthesized in the liver to produce steroidal hormones. High cholesterol in the bloodstream virtually translates into high levels of DHT as well.

Our diet is also low in fiber, which means that foods abide in our systems longer than they should. The food ferments as a result of increased bacteria, augmenting the toxicity levels in the bloodstream, and further inhibiting the optimal absorption of nutrients.The bottom line is that the hair follicles rely on the nutrients they receive from the blood. Insufficient quantities of fiber are another key factor in inhibiting hair growth.

With the understanding that hair is 97 percent protein, it is easy to see how insufficient levels of protein intake can also be a contributing component in hair loss and poor hair health. Strict vegetarians, vegans, people on severe weight-loss regimens, and those suffering from eating disorders (*i.e.*, anorexia nervosa or bulimia) do not ingest an adequate daily supply of protein. Hair loss usually begins within two to three months as the follicles in the growth cycle shift into the dormant telogen state in a defensive attempt to conserve protein levels.

Before you jump to the conclusion that increasing protein levels to high amounts will prevent hair loss, you should know that eating too much protein will cause the same problems as eating too little. If protein intake exceeds 15 to 20 percent of your diet, your body will go into a kind of "negative mineral balance" and react virtually the same as when protein levels are inadequate. Daily protein intake should never exceed more than 30 to 40 grams.

Studies have also linked salt intake to hair loss. Sodium from common table salt is retained in the tissues of the scalp (and throughout the body), hampering their functions.

A nutritionally balanced diet will not be of much benefit if the body is incapable of transmuting the elements it requires. As we get older, the body is less and less able to absorb nutrients. This is initially indicated by the fact that the stomach fails to produce as much acid as it did earlier in life, evidenced by the increased presence of gas, heartburn, and bloating. Sensations of exhaustion after a meal tend to point to the digestion process also burning up too much energy.

Protein, which is the building block of hair, is usually the first victim of poor digestion.

Proper digestion involves four principal stages, and begins in the mouth with the production of saliva. Saliva launches the digestive course by breaking down carbohydrates and preparing food for peristalsis, the journey through the digestive tract. The secretion of stomach acids is activated by the chewing action.

The second stage happens in the stomach with the secretion of enzymes from the pancreas. These enzymes break down the food, and are replaced from enzymes found *only* in raw foods. Since the quintessential Western diet accentuates cooked foods over raw, the pancreas is frequently unable to secrete adequate levels of enzymes by middle age, and requires the assistance of an enzyme supplement. Ironically, while a supplement will assist the pancreas, it will also weaken it by making it dependent on the supplement.

The third stage involves the secretion of hydrochloric acid to further the breakdown of food. Heartburn results from an insufficient level of this acid.

When the food is almost completely digested, it passes from the stomach into the intestines. Stage four involves the bacteria *acidophilus*, which plays a large part in enzyme production and conveys nutrients into the bloodstream. Acidophilus also supports the immune system, coordinates oscillations in hormone levels, controls the amounts of cholesterol, and is a preventative factor in cancer of the colon.

Unfortunately, acidophilus is easily annihilated by many factors in our diet and culture. Chlorinated tap water, food poisoning, and smoking are just a few. Antibiotics, which are intended to kill bacteria, act haphazard in their task, killing the helpful acidophilus bacteria without differentiation. Insufficient levels of acidophilus give rise to harmful bacteria, essentially poisoning the bloodstream. Classic symptoms of low acidophilus levels include increased flatulence, halitosis (bad breath), acne, indigestion, and headaches. (Food products such as yogurt, miso, and sourdough do contain acidophilus, but in such insufficient levels that they fail to have any restorative function. Concentrated acidophilus in the refrigerator section of your supermarket or health food store is the only thing that will rebuild this bacterium in your system.)

The high fat/high protein composition of most Western diets leads to a buildup of fatty deposits along the walls of the intestinal tract, effectively preventing the absorption of nutrients into the bloodstream. As the buildup continues over time and the body becomes increasingly deprived of vitamins and minerals, the feeling of satisfaction after a meal becomes more and more difficult to achieve.

To discharge this buildup, an increase of fiber is necessary. Psyllium husks do the trick quite well, and are commonly found in such commercial products as Metamucil. Psyllium husks inflate with water and scour the intestinal walls, pushing out old matter. Since it will also indiscriminately remove bacteria, an acidophilus supplement should be taken along with psyllium husks. A cleansing program of one level tablespoon of psyllium husks mixed with six ounces of water (accompanied by another six ounces of water with acidophilus) twice daily can be implemented for up to ten days. Thereafter, once or twice a week should be sufficient.

Vitamins in adequate measures are absolutely indispensable to maintaining the health of the body. The condition and quantity of hair on the scalp is a direct reflection of that vitality. While it is outside the range of this book to be the definitive guide on the general well-being of the body, it is pertinent to look at the vitamins and minerals that are closely connected to preventing hair loss, stimulating growth, and engendering healthy hair. You should keep in mind that your nutritional requirements will be particular to your age, weight, height, diet, etc. It is recommended that you consult a nutritional specialist or your physician before taking a trip to the health food store to buy up an inventory of supplements. We will also be suggesting dietary changes that should more than adequately meet your needs.

Vitamin A is essential for strong bones, sharp eyes, healthy glands, skin, teeth, and hair. When combined with zinc and silica, it assists in the proper functioning of the sebaceous glands. Vitamin A deficiencies can lead to a clogging of the sebaceous glands and a thickening of the scalp, which symptomatically leads to flaking and a buildup of sebum in the pores. With the pores closed off, the follicles cannot breathe, and hair cannot grow.

Smoking, air pollution, aspirin products, antibiotics, laxatives, barbiturates, and certain cholesterol-lowering drugs can work to deplete the body of vitamin A. Ten thousand IU per day is considered a safe supplemental dosage for most adults. This vitamin is fat-soluble, which means the body stores whatever it doesn't immediately use in fat cells (unlike B and C vitamins, which are water-soluble with the excess being eliminated through urine). Too high of a dosage of vitamin A can inflame the hair follicles, so it's very important not to overdo it.

Foods that are rich in vitamin A:

Alfalfa	Celery	Parsley
Apricots	Fish liver oils	Rose hips
Beets	Green and red peppers	Sweet potatoes
Broccoli	Liver	Spinach (organic)
Cabbage	Kale	Tomatoes
Cantaloupe	Oranges	Yellow squash
Carrots		Watercress

A good general rule of thumb to follow is: if it's a yellow or green fruit or vegetable, then it's probably high in vitamin A.

The B-complex of vitamins has gained a lot of notoriety for its ability to impact the health of hair. It should be noted that the Bs are interconnected and depend upon one another to have any useful effect on the body. While a number of specific Bs play a significant role in the health and growth of your hair, you should always take a B-complex. You can, of course, augment the intake of particular Bs known to stimulate hair growth and vitality, but they should never be taken on their own. They just won't work without the entire B-complex family.

Foods that are rich in B-complex vitamins:
Cucumber
Dark leafy vegetables

One of those Bs, biotin, has particularly been touted for its preventative properties in hair loss. It works as a coenzyme that aids in the proper absorption of carbohydrates, fats, and proteins; and supports cell growth, the assimilation of essential fatty acids, and assists the body in the employment of other B vitamins. Biotin has a high sulfur content, which is a mineral the body uses as a primary cleansing agent, and is an indispensable component for stimulating hair growth. Sulfur comprises about 0.25 percent of the body, and can be found in every cell, with the highest concentrations found in hair, skin, and nails. It detoxifies the blood and protects against radiation and pollution. Sulfur is a key component of the protein structure keratin, which comprises 97 percent of the hair shaft.

Considerable evidence has also shown that biotin, when used topically with niacin (a form of B-3 that releases histamines), does promote hair growth.

Grain alcohol, antibiotics, and egg whites are known to nullify biotin. A good supplemental dosage is about 300 micrograms, but should be taken with a B-complex to promote absorption and balance the body's usage of the Bs.

Foods that are rich in biotin:

Brewer's yeast	Kidney	Poultry
Brown rice	Lettuce	Seafood
Cauliflower	Liver	Soybeans
Egg yolk	Mushrooms	Spinach (organic)
Grapefruit	Nutritional yeast	

Foods that are rich in sulfur:

Brussels sprouts	Dried beans	Fish
Cabbage	Egg yolk	Turnips

Niacin, a form of vitamin B-3, works wonders in stimulating blood circulation. At a dosage of about 100 mg, niacin taken on its own (which is the only exception in the B-complex family) will release histamines in the body, flushing blood to the capillaries throughout the skin, including the scalp. If you've never taken a niacin supplement, you should know that the release of histamines will cause a distinct tingling sensation, and your skin will temporarily turn red with a slight rash. This is completely normal and harmless. Additionally, the release of histamines will also discharge heparin, a substance which is essential for cell growth and is intimately connected to the papilla's production of hair cells.

Niacin is also marketed in a formula with 200 micrograms of chromium, which is taken for lowering cholesterol and does not have the tingling side effect. *Do not buy this version*, as it is only possible to obtain the histamine-releasing properties when niacin is taken on its own.

There are two members of the B-complex family that specifically work as antioxidants and as cell membrane stabilizers: inositol, and para-aminobenzoic acid (commonly known as PABA). These two vitamins have a shielding action on the hair follicles by protecting them from membrane damage promoted by oxidized cholesterol collecting in the scalp.

PABA behaves as a coenzyme, assisting in breaking down proteins in the bloodstream and utilizing them efficiently. It is also a key supporting factor in the healthy production of red blood cells. Studies with daily doses of 1,000 to 3,000 mg have indicated that PABA does retard hair loss and reverses premature graying of the hair stemming from nutritional deficiencies and stress. It is usually recommended in doses of 100 mg in a healthy dietary regimen.

Foods that are rich in PABA:		
Cabbage	Nutritional yeast	Spinach (organic)
Eggs	Oats	Sunflower seeds
Mushrooms		Whole grains

By linking with choline to form lecithin, inositol stimulates a healthful stream of nutrients and blood flowing to the hair follicles and scalp region. Similar to PABA, studies have demonstrated that inositol is connected to the prevention of hair loss and premature graying. Because of its link to the formation of lecithin, it also works at metabolizing cholesterol and fats, and prevents the narrowing and hardening of the arteries. Inositol is also noted for its sedative effects, and can be used to alleviate mild cases of hypertension by lowering blood pressure.

In cases of hair loss related to stress, inositol plays a major role in treatment. Symptoms of an inositol deficiency besides hair loss include abnormalities of the eyes, eczema, constipation, and insomnia. Those who drink black tea, coffee, and sodas with caffeine should be aware that caffeine depletes the body of inositol, and should therefore consider cutting back on their consumption and/or taking a supplement. Recommended daily doses range from 100 to 200 mg in your dietary regimen.

Foods that are rich in inositol:

Kale	Oranges
Lecithin	Tomatoes
Legumes	Unrefined molasses
Nutritional yeast	Whole grains
Onions	

Far more notable for its antistress properties than inositol is B-5, pantothenic acid. In fact, B-5 has gained so much credibility for stress reduction that it is commonly marketed as the primary ingredient in antistress vitamin formulas. B-5 also plays a primary part in producing adrenal hormones, and it is an essential vitamin in the output of antibodies. It also serves the body in assimilating many other vitamins, and the efficient metabolizing of proteins, fats, and carbohydrates. Symptoms of B-5 deficiency can include hypoglycemia, fatigue, irritability, skin problems, premature aging, as well as hair loss and premature graying. Pantothenic acid has also been used in the treatment of depression and some anxiety disorders. Remarkably, there is evidence that this vitamin also extends life expectancy, having demonstrated a 20 percent increase in the life expectancy of lab mice, while augmenting endurance and stamina. For hair loss prevention, recommended daily supplemental dosages are 100 mg taken three times daily.

Foods that are rich in B-5:

Beans	Fresh vegetables	Oranges
Bee pollen	Grapefruit	Royal jelly
Cauliflower	L-cysteine	Saltwater fish
Eggs		Strawberries

L-cysteine is an amino acid that comprises approximately 8 percent of hair, and is commonly included as a component in many hair growth vitamin supplements. It works to preserve and protect cells by combating harmful toxins in the bloodstream. High doses of L-cysteine can reverse the positive effects of this amino acid, and can lead to bladder or kidney stones. When taking L-cysteine, it is strongly recommended that three times as much vitamin C be ingested along with it, since vitamin C counteracts the toxic effects of high levels of L-cysteine. A hair growth regimen should include 500 mg of L-cysteine accompanied by at least 1,500 mg of vitamin C two times per day.

Foods that are rich in L-cysteine:		
Alfalfa	Carrots	Horseradish
Apples	Cauliflower	Kale
Beets	Currants	Legumes
Brussels sprouts	Filberts	Onions
Cabbage	Garlic	Pineapples
	Hazelnuts	

Vitamins C and E are also critical to hair growth. Vitamin C performs a multitude of functions throughout the body. It is a significant factor in the formation of collagen, is obligatory for proper adrenal gland functions (indispensable in managing stress levels), and encourages healthy circulation to the scalp. Recommended daily dosages for hair growth range from 500 to 3,000 mg in a time-released formula. Check to make sure that the vitamin C supplement you purchase includes bioflavinoids, which are a cofactor for the proper absorption of vitamin C and work to reinforce the capillaries and veins all through the bloodstream (including the ones feeding the papilla in your scalp).

Foods that are rich in vitamin C:		
Black currants	Green peppers	Parsley
Cabbage	Kale	Rose hips
Citrus fruits		Spinach (organic)

Increasing oxygen intake to the bloodstream is of vital necessity for improving circulation in the scalp, and this is the role of vitamin E. Deficiencies in vitamin E are indicated by brittle, dull hair shafts, as well as hair loss. A hair growth program should include between 400 IU to 800 IU of *natural* vitamin E. (Avoid the synthetic versions derived from petroleum, as the body does have a problem absorbing it, and eventually blocks it at the E receptor sites.)

Foods that are rich in vitamin E:
Cold-pressed vegetable oils, especially wheat germ oil

Here's a summary table of the vitamins discussed here and their cofactors, showing the foods they can be found in:

Vitamins	Foods
A	(Occurs in nature only as carotene, which is converted in the body to Vitamin A.) Alfalfa, apricots, beets, broccoli, cantaloupe, carrots, cabbage, celery, fish liver oils, green and red peppers, kale, liver, parsley, oranges and rose hips, spinach, sweet potatoes, tomatoes, yellow squash, watercress

Vitamins	Foods
B-complex	Cucumbers, dark leafy vegetables
B-1	Beet tops, beets, carrots, dandelion, grapefruit, spinach
B-2	Beet tops, carrots, celery, green peppers, kale, parsley, spinach, turnip greens
B-3 (Niacin)	Asparagus, kale, parsley, potatoes
B-5	Beans, bee pollen, cabbage, cauliflower, eggs, fresh vegetables, grapefruit, oranges, royal jelly, saltwater fish, strawberries
B-6	Carrots, lemons, pears, potatoes, spinach
Folic Acid	Carrots, oranges, parsley, potatoes, spinach
Biotin	Brewer's yeast, brown rice, cauliflower, egg yolk, grapefruit, kidney, lettuce, liver, mushrooms, nutritional yeast, poultry, seafood, soybeans, spinach
PABA	Cabbage, eggs, mushrooms, nutritional yeast, oats, spinach, sunflower seeds, whole grains
Inositol	Beets, cabbage, cauliflower, citrus fruits, kale, lecithin, legumes, nutritional yeast, onions, oranges, tomatoes, unrefined molasses, whole grains
C	Black currants, cabbage, citrus fruits, green peppers, kale, parsley, rose hips, spinach
L-Cysteine	Alfalfa, apples, beets, brussels sprouts, cabbage, carrots, cauliflower, currants, filberts, garlic, hazelnuts, horseradish, kale, legumes, onions, pineapples
E	Cold-pressed vegetable oils, especially wheat germ

Along with the vitamins listed previously, there are a number of essential minerals that are required for your hair's roots to take in proper nourishment: iodine, zinc (especially for men), sulfur (which we've discussed), potassium, iron, and silica.

Iodine regulates the thyroid gland, encouraging the hormone thyroxin. Thyroxin metabolizes and conveys nutrients to the millions of blood vessels, nerve endings, and lymph vessels throughout the body, as well as all of the sebaceous glands in your scalp. Thyroxin passes through the subcutaneous layer of fat just under the scalp and feeds the hair follicles, inducing the sebaceous glands to secrete sebum. The most effective iodine supplement available is made from sea kelp and other ocean plants. This form of iodine is chemically indistinguishable from the form located in the thyroid gland. It is also recommended that you switch from common iodized table salt to noniodized sea salt. Iodized table salt is a synthetic form of iodine, which builds up in the body and eventually overwhelms the thyroid.

Zinc deficiencies can also inhibit the hormonal functions of the thyroid. It should be noted that most American men are zinc deficient. Deficiencies are often linked to having too much copper in your environment, especially hot-water plumbing, cookware, or some contraceptive devices for women. Studies have shown that zinc improves the body's ability to utilize vitamin A. Since these two work so well together, it is logical that your program should include both; 3 mg of copper should also be taken, as it supports the body's metabolic absorption of zinc.

Recommended daily zinc dosages range from 15 mg to 50 mg. However, taking too much zinc can also inhibit the thyroid. Since each body has different needs, you must be careful when taking a zinc supplement. Zinc cannot be tasted when the body is deficient, but it has a distinct metallic taste when enough has been absorbed. Purchase a nonflavored zinc lozenge with a low potency of about 5 mg per tablet. Keep track of how many lozenges you ingest by starting with three 5 mg tablets, and gradually increase the amount over a few days. At some point you will notice the taste change, and that means you've exceeded your maximum. Zinc is stored in the body, so reduce your intake a bit over the next few days until the metallic flavor has disappeared. At that point, you need to begin increasing the dosage again.

Foods that are rich in zinc:

Egg yolks	Nutritional yeast	Soybeans
Fish	Oats	Spinach (steamed)
Legumes	Pumpkin seeds	Sunflower seeds
Mushrooms	Seafood (especially oysters)	Tomatoes (raw)

Potassium promotes optimal muscle contraction and, along with sodium, balances the levels of water retained by the body. (Diuretic drugs and caffeine can easily deplete potassium.) Potassium also plays a role in distributing nutrients throughout the body and is essential in hormonal secretions. Symptoms of potassium deficiency include persistent fatigue, dull or lackluster hair, eczema, itchy scalp, and a condition in which the hair oscillates from being extremely oily to being extremely dry.

Foods that are rich in potassium:

Avocados	Kale	Parsley
Bananas	Lemons	Potatoes
Celery	Molasses	Spinach
Dried fruits	Nutritional yeast	Tangerines
Grapes	Nuts	Yams

Symptoms of a low-grade iron deficiency include dry, brittle hair, as well as fatigue and rough, chapped skin. Full-blown anemia is often indicated by hair loss. If you suspect that you have anemia or may be iron deficient, *it is strongly recommended that you consult your doctor.* When purchasing an iron supplement, avoid the common type called ferrous sulfate. It is remarkably difficult for the body to assimilate, often building up deposits in the liver and eventually leading to serious liver problems. Before taking an iron supplement, you should try correcting the deficiency by adjusting your diet.

Foods that are rich in iron:

Almonds	Eggs	Molasses
Beets	Fish	Poultry
Dates	Green leafy vegetables	Raisins
Dried prunes	Kidney and lima beans	Whole grains

Oxygen is the most abundant element on the earth. Silicon is the second, and is encountered chiefly in the form of silica. Silica promotes cell metabolism and production, controlling the aging process. It maintains and restores our eyes, teeth, nails, skin, and hair. A silica supplement should only be purchased if it has been processed as an "organic vegetal silica from aqueous extract."

Unprocessed silica is usually sold in the herb horsetail. *Ingesting unprocessed horsetail can have extremely toxic side effects, particularly on the prostate gland in men.* Recommended daily dosages of an aqueous silica extract supplement range from 10 to 20 mg. For hair restoration, daily dosages should be increased to levels between 30 and 60 mg for up to one month.

Foods that are rich in silica:		
Asparagus	Leeks	Rhubarb
Cabbage	Lettuce	Rice, Rice, Rice
Cauliflower	Oats	Strawberries
Celery	Onions	Sunflower seeds
Cucumber	Parsnip	Swiss chard

Another interesting note about silica is that it is found in exceptional amounts in nettles, which is a factor that accounts for this plant's restorative properties in hair. Organic vegetal silica can be purchased in a powder form and added to any of the shampoo recipes in Chapter Seven. (There are a few commercial shampoos available that include silica as an ingredient, but the amount is insufficient to have any effect; it's not much more than a clever ploy from the manufacturer's marketing department.)

Here's a summary table of the minerals discussed here, and some of their cofactors, showing the foods they can be found in:

Minerals	Foods
Calcium	Cabbage, carrots, elderberries, kale, lemons, milk, mustard greens, tangerines, turnips, watercress
Iron	Almonds, beets, dates, dried prunes, eggs, fish, green leafy vegetables, kidney and lima beans, molasses, poultry, raisins, whole grains
Magnesium	Beets, elderberries, endive, lemons, raspberries
Phosphorous	Beet tops, cabbage, carrots, grapes, kale, raspberries, spinach, tangerines, watercress
Potassium	Avocados, bananas, celery, dandelions, dried fruits, grapes, kale, lemons, molasses, nutritional yeast, nuts, parsley, potatoes, spinach, tangerines, yams, most leafy green vegetables
Silica	Asparagus, cabbage, cauliflower, celery, cucumber, leeks, lettuce, oats, onions, parsnip, rhubarb, rice, strawberries, sunflower seeds, Swiss chard
Sodium	Beets, carrots, celery, cherries, dandelions, kale, peaches, tomatoes
Sulfur	Brussels sprouts, cabbage, dried beans, egg yolk, fish, turnips
Zinc	Egg yolks, fish, legumes, mushrooms, nutritional yeast, oats, pumpkin seeds, seafood (especially oysters), soybeans, spinach, sunflower seeds, tomatoes (raw)

When most of us think of supplements, we think only of vitamins and minerals. But we're missing out on a vital third class known as Essential Fatty Acids (EFAs). EFAs assist in maintaining the well-being of the body, mind, and emotions, and are considered essential for your diet because they are not naturally produced in the body. Low level deficiencies are indicated by dry, brittle hair, hair loss, and skin (which also includes the scalp) conditions of dryness, flaking, itching, or psoriasis. Advanced occurrences of EFA deficiencies include symptoms of confusion, fatigue, general weakness, bruising, pain, and inflammation in the joints. There is also convincing evidence in recent medical studies that EFA deficiencies lead to a swelling of the sebaceous glands, giving rise to excessive secretions of sebum. In turn, this incites clogging of the follicles, malnutrition of the hair root, and increased hormone levels of 5-alpha reductase (which is converted into DHT, restricts vasodilation to the papilla, and advances hair loss).

Supplemental sources of EFA are available in cod liver oil, wheat germ oil, evening primrose oil, and flaxseed oil. Avoid taking cod liver oil, since the amount required for any therapeutic benefit is so great that you will run a grave risk of overdosing on vitamins A and D.

Evening primrose and flaxseed oils are available in capsule and liquid forms. They each have slightly different fatty acids, so they should *both* be included in your daily regimen. Normal dosages should be three capsules, or one tablespoon of each per day. For hair growth and restoration, the amounts should be doubled to six capsules, or two tablespoons of each per day. Since these fatty acids lack certain cofactors required to derive their benefits, you must take them along with a good multivitamin and mineral supplement. Make sure the following nutrients are included: biotin, niacin, B-6, C, E, and zinc.

High levels of saturated fats found in vegetable and animal products work against EFAs, so avoid taking these supplements with meals prepared using those fats. Additional things to avoid that could hinder the body's absorption of EFAs are: high cholesterol levels, immoderate alcohol consumption, diabetes, repeated viral infections, and nutritional deficiencies. Unavoidably, old age also hinders the assimilation of EFAs. Consuming polyunsaturated fatty acids (hydrogenated vegetable oils, like margarine and deep fried foods) will also stop EFAs in their tracks. (Polyunsaturated fatty acids are a chief ingredient in the formation of free radicals in the body, and should be avoided at all costs. Free radicals are now commonly believed to be the mechanism responsible for premature aging, problems with the immune system, and cancer.)

Because of this, it is highly recommended that you refrain from cooking with vegetable oils, shortening, and animal fats. Replace them with monounsaturated fats such as olive, canola, and peanut oils. These oils do not interfere with EFAs, nor do they promote free radicals. Your palate may need to adjust to the tastes produced from cooking with these oils, but they are lighter and allow for the true flavors of the foods to come through in their preparation.

An excellent source for EFAs is deep-sea fish such as salmon, mackerel, trout, herring, or sardines. Two or three meals a week including one of these should provide an adequate supply of EFAs.

There are a number of herbs that are known for their ability to improve the condition of the scalp and promote hair growth. One of these, nettles, has already been mentioned repeatedly through this book. An extract derived from nettle root has been successfully shown to inhibit the activity of 5-alpha reductase, as well as bolstering the endocrine glands. (In men, nettle root extract also works as a decongestive on the prostate gland, relieving discomfort from conditions of enlargement.)

Saw palmetto has gained an even more substantial reputation than that of nettles. An extract derived from serenoa repens (saw palmetto berries) is effective at blocking the conversion of testosterone into DHT, and also prevents DHT's ability to lock onto cellular receptor sites. A recommended dose of saw palmetto extract is 160 mg taken twice a day.

Foenumgraecum, commonly known as fenugreek, is a plant widely used for a variety of medicinal applications. The seeds are very nourishing, and are customarily administered to convalescing patients to encourage weight gain, especially those suffering from anorexia nervosa. Fenugreek also helps to inhibit cancer of the liver, lower blood cholesterol levels, and is used as an antidiabetic. It works in combination with thyme as a strong mucilage that cleans the mucous from the body, maximizing the metabolic synthesis of vitamins, minerals, EFAs, and other herbs, making it indispensable for a hair-growth or hair-restoration program. Crushed seeds can also be mixed with olive oil and massaged into the hair to give it a glossy sheen.

Here's a table of other herbs and plants that are effective in the care of your hair. Take this list to your local herbal supply or health food store and ask your supplier to recommend the best brands and combinations available:

Dark hair	Bergamot, clove, creosote, jaborandi, nettle, rosemary, sage, southernwood
Dry hair	Acacia, chamomile, clover, comfrey root, cowslip, elderflower, melitot, orange flower, peach leaf
Eczema	Burdock, cade, germander, lycopodium powder, moss, pansy, pine tar, thyme, violet, white willow bark
Hair conditioning	Basil oil, cherry bark, lavender oil, nettle and cherry bark, ragwort, rosemary
Hair growth	American bearsfoot, astralgus root, butcher's brood, ginger and horseradish, gingko biloba leaves, jaborandi, marshmallow root, rhubarb root, rosemary, sea kelp, shave grass, southernwood, spirulina, uva ursi
Hair loss	Ginger and horseradish, gobernadora, rosemary, shave grass, southernwood, spirulina
Light hair	Chamomile, comfrey root, cowslip flower, elderflower, marigold, orrisroot, quassia chip, white willow bark
Oily hair	Bergamot, lemongrass, orrisroot, quassia chip, strawberry, white willow bark, witch hazel bark
Psoriasis	Birch bark, chamomile, cajuput, comfrey root, germander, lecithin, pansy, papaya, sea kelp, thyme, white willow bark, wintergreen

Supplement Summary

For your convenience, here is a summary listing of the major points in this chapter, with all the vitamins, minerals, and EFAs described, as well as others that work in concert with them. Take this list to your local health food store, and read the labels on the supplement bottles. If you have any questions, talk to the person behind the counter. You will be surprised to find how well informed they are. Western culture has begun to acknowledge the healing powers of herbs and other supplements, and the people who work in health food stores have had to become highly proficient in the subtleties of how these supplements work.

Protein Intake: 30 to 40 grams per day (or 15 to 20 percent of your diet)

Psyllium Husks: (always taken with an acidophilus supplement)

Cleansing Program: one level tablespoon mixed in 6 ounces of water, and an acidophilus supplement with an additional 6 ounces of water twice daily for up to 10 days.

Maintenance Program: one level tablespoon mixed in 6 ounces of water, and an acidophilus supplement with an additional 6 ounces of water twice a week.

Vitamins

- Vitamin A: 10,000 IU per day
- A good B-complex should include the following:
  - B-3 (niacin in a B-complex supplement): 50 mg three times per day
  - B-3 (niacin by itself *without chromium or any other supplements*): for stimulation of hair growth, take 100 mg once daily
  - B-5: 100 mg three times per day
  - B-6: 50 mg three times per day
  - Biotin: 100 mg three times per day
  - Folic Acid: 100 mg three times per day

- Inositol: 100 to 200 mg per day
- PABA: 100 mg per day (for hair loss: 1,000 to 3,000 mg per day)
- L-cysteine: 500 mg twice per day *with 1,500 mg of vitamin C at each dosage.*
- Vitamin E *(natural only; avoid petroleum-derived versions)*: 400 to 800 IU per day.

Minerals
- Copper: 3 mg per day
- Iodine: 150 mg per day
- Iron: *Use only with a doctor's supervision.*
- Sea Kelp: 500 mg per day
- Potassium: 200 mg per day
- Selenium: 30 mg per day
- Silica (purchase only versions derived as "organic vegetal silica from aqueous extract"): take 10 to 20 mg daily; for hair growth stimulation, increase to between 30 and 40 mg per day
- Zinc: use 5 mg lozenges ranging between 15 to 50 mg daily, depending upon the presence of a metallic taste

Essential Fatty Acids (EFAs)
- Evening Primrose Oil and Flaxseed Oil: 3 capsules or 1 tablespoon of each once per day; for hair growth stimulation, take 6 capsules or 2 tablespoons of each once per day

Hair Growth Protein Shake
I recommend that you have this delicious protein shake every day. You can vary the flavor by changing the fruit you're using. It's

satisfying and delicious, and provides your body with many nutrients that support hair growth.

Hair Growth Protein Shake

1 tablespoon whey or soy protein

8 ounces pure water

Fresh fruit (blueberries, half of a banana, etc.)

1 tablespoon lecithin

1 tablespoon brewer's yeast

1 tablespoon flaxseed oil

8-10 kelp tablets (optional)

Put all ingredients into blender and blend until smooth. Add ice cubes if desired.

Hair Growth and Restoration Diet

A lot of options and information have so far been included in this chapter. It might be helpful for you to tie it all together with a suggested diet that will revitalize your body and stimulate the growth and luster of your hair. This diet really should be considered more as a guideline than something to be used as a strict regimen to punish yourself with. As long as you stick with the foods mentioned in this chapter, and follow the principles of good nutrition, you will find that you have a lot of room to eat satisfying foods in satisfying portions.

Here are a few things to remember when making food choices:

- Drink water, *lots* of water—at least 8 ounces an hour.
- Cut down on caffeine intake or eliminate it altogether.

- If you must use a sweetener for your coffee, tea, or just about anything else, try to use a substitute. At the very least, use brown or raw sugar.
- Cut down on your intake of table salt, preferably cutting it out all together.
- Eliminate alcoholic beverages.
- Start out your program with a psyllium husk cleanser, twice a day for the first 7 to 10 days. Thereafter, take a maintenance dose once or twice a week. You can mix it in juice or a protein shake. Remember to take an acidophilus supplement to restore those critical enzymes.
- Stick to fresh foods. Steam your vegetables for no more than 5 minutes. Refrain from processed or refined products, particularly jellies and sweets.
- Remove any fat and skin from all meats before preparing.
- If you take vitamin supplements, take them at the *end* of the meal, unless the instructions specifically say otherwise.
- Cut out the polyunsaturated fats, like vegetable oils, margarine, and animal fats from your diet. Cook with monounsaturated fats such as olive, canola, and peanut oils. These oils do not interfere with EFAs, nor do they promote free radicals.
- If you're a vegetarian or wish to cut back on your intake of meat, you will need to get your protein from other sources. Combining certain food groups in your recipes and cooking will optimize your selections:
   - Grains (cereals, corn, pasta, or rice) can be combined with legumes (beans, lentils, or peas).

- Grains can be combined with dairy products such as cheese and milk.
- Seeds (sesame or sunflower) can be combined with legumes.

Here are some specific food choice guidelines that are proven to stimulate hair growth:

- Avoid dairy products, including: milk, cream, cheese, cottage cheese, yogurt, butter, ice cream, and any products that are made with casein.
- Choose chicken, turkey, lamb, and fish over beef, pork, or veal.
- Choose gluten-free products such as those made from rice, millet, buckwheat, and gluten-free flour. Avoid wheat, spelt, kamut, oat, rye, barley, and malt.
- Avoid yeast or foods that promote yeast overgrowth. This includes refined sugars, condiments, fermented foods, and peanuts.

Here is how to make the most of the food groups:

- *Meat, Fish, Poultry, Legumes, Eggs:* The best foods in this group are chicken, turkey, lamb, salmon, halibut, mackerel, trout, dried peas, lentils, and egg substitutes.
- *Dairy:* Choose milk substitutes such as rice or soy milk.
- *Starches:* Potatoes, sweet potatoes, arrowroot, rice, tapioca, buckwheat, or millet. Avoid gluten.
- *Bread/Cereal:* Choose those made from rice, quinoa, amaranth, buckwheat, teff, millet, soy, potato flour, tapioca, arrowroot, or gluten-free flour.

- *Vegetables:* All vegetables are good choices, especially fresh or frozen.
- *Fruit:* Fresh fruit is also a good choice (with no sweeteners). Avoid citrus and strawberries.
- *Fats/Oils:* Canola, flax, olive, pumpkin, sesame, and walnut oils are best. Avoid margarine, shortening, butter, and refined oils.
- *Nuts/Seeds:* Almonds, cashews, pecans, walnuts, pumpkin seeds, sesame seeds, squash, flax or sunflower seeds, as well as nut butters made from any of these. Avoid peanuts, pistachios, and peanut butter.
- *Sweeteners:* Brown rice syrup or fruit sweeteners are best, avoid white and brown sugar, honey, molasses, corn syrup, and fructose.

Pull out your recipe books, get creative, and have fun! Cooking can relieve a lot of stress and promote a positive sense of well-being.

14

The Importance of Exercise

Increasing the flow of oxygen to the bloodstream is a primary goal in any hair growth and restoration program. Exercise is an important component in achieving that goal. It should be an essential part of anyone's lifestyle, not merely because of its widely recognized benefits—weight control, improved cardiovascular fitness, increased strength, protection against diabetes, and an improved sense of well-being—but with regards to the subject at hand, you should be aware that exercise, or the lack of it, has a significant impact on the adrenal system throughout the body. In short, the adrenal glands and hormonal secretions of a sedentary person do not function as optimally as do those of someone who exercises regularly. Another benefit is the fact that vigorous exercise will also release hormonal eicosanoids, which dilate the blood vessels and increase the flow of oxygen to the capillaries (including those feeding the follicles in the scalp).

Clearly the goals of increasing the flow of oxygen to the bloodstream and decreasing the body's fat content are of paramount concern to someone seeking to stimulate hair growth or restore vitality to hair.

To receive the benefits of stimulating hair growth, you will need to perform some type of vigorous activity for a minimum of

20 to 60 minutes, three to four times a week. This vigorous activity must be executed nonstop at between 60 percent and 80 percent of your Maximum Heart Rate (MHR).

Your Maximum Heart Rate (MHR)

What is your Maximum Heart Rate? It can be determined with a calculator and the following formula:
1. Subtract your current age from 220. This number is your MHR.
2. Multiply this number by 0.60. This is 60 percent of your MHR.
3. Take the number you came up with in Step 1. Multiply it by 0.80. This is 80 percent of your MHR.

These numbers of 60 percent and 80 percent represent the range of your Target Heart Rate (THR). (An important note: many high blood pressure medications work by lowering the heart rate, which would mean that your MHR and target rates may need to be lowered as well. If you are taking any blood pressure medications, contact your physician to find out how best to adjust these numbers.)

When engaging in exercise, you will need to keep track of your heart rate to make sure you are staying within the 60 percent to 80 percent THR range. This is commonly done by lightly pressing the index finger of the right hand over the artery just under the skin on the inside of the left wrist. The rate is easily determined by counting the beats for 15 seconds, then multiplying that number by a factor of 4. This will be your heart rate. (If you can't do the math in your head while working out, then try counting the beats for an entire minute.)

If you don't like the idea of measuring your pulse while working out, there is an alternative rule of thumb: if you can hold a conversation, you aren't working hard enough. If you can sing, you're not working hard enough either. If you are out of breath, or have to stop and catch your breath, you're definitely working too hard.

Most people connect the idea of exercise with being miserable. Getting up at 5:30 to jog down a cold, foggy highway, or to pedal for a long, boring hour on a squeaky stationary bike immediately comes to mind. Let's be honest here: these forms of exercise are not natural. (Of course, if you love to jog or ride a stationary bike, by all means keep it up!) The point here is that the human body was designed for movement, and movement should be enjoyed as much as any other form of sensory stimulation. If jogging and riding stationary bikes seem like disagreeable and unpleasant forms of movement to you, then forget about them.

The human body was engineered for physical motion: walking, dancing, biking, playing games, and playing with children. These activities can get your circulation going and your body will derive many benefits, but don't we really do those things for the fun of it? The point here is that moving your body should be as enjoyable as anything else you choose to do.

Start your program with very simple activities. Take a walk in the woods, or walk the neighborhood 30 to 60 minutes, three times per week. Find a place to walk that is agreeable and pleasant for you. If you prefer, choose any of these other activities:

Bicycling	Jumping rope	Swimming
Canoeing	Racquetball	Tennis (singles)
Dancing		Volleyball

For people who can't engage in vigorous exercise, there is a lot of evidence that even moderately intense activities will bring about good health benefits. These activities can include:

Gardening	Ping-Pong	Touch football
Golf	Tennis (doubles)	Walking for pleasure
Housework		Yard work

These are just a few ideas intended to get you thinking. Feel free to come up with your own. The key is to stay in vigorous motion for at least 20 to 60 minutes three to four times a week, and to make it fun.

On the other end of the spectrum, while excess body fat is bothersome to your health, having too little is just as bad, if not worse. A

(BMI) number below 25 can wreak havoc with the immune system, cause fatigue, and interrupt menstrual regularity and estrogen levels in women. It is also a cause of hair loss.

If you are overweight or underweight, start by seeing your physician, and perhaps a professional trainer for guidance. Every step counts in restoring your hair, and this one is no less important.

15

In Conclusion

Many clients who walk through the doors of *Riquette International* come with a deep sense of anguish, fear, and frustration over the condition of their hair. Their stories are fraught with a great deal of pain and anger, and are often profound in their shame and loss of hope. Our task in repairing the health of our client's hair is never just about the scalp. It also requires compassion, understanding, and a heartfelt commitment to recuperating their lost sense of self-esteem. Our work is only complete when joy, vitality, and pride have been healed.

Trust. Love. Integrity. Peace These are the four elements we work with and strive to instill in our clients. The men, women, and children who come to us must learn to trust that there is hope, and that they have not reached the end of the line, so to speak. They must have compassion for themselves by releasing the fear and anger; this is an act of self-love. Most clients look in the mirror, see only their hair loss and damage, and believe that they are flawed. The mirror doesn't reveal the truth that they are every bit as lovable as the day they were born. We teach them to look deeper, beyond the brutal reality of their condition, to see the essence of their spirit. As it says in the ancient Vedic scriptures of the *Bhagavad Gita*, "Life is love, and love is life. What keeps the body together but love?"

While trust and love are the foundation of the program, the promise of restored vitality and health can only be fulfilled by following each step with absolute integrity, the third element. A rigorous adherence to the coaching and guidelines set forth in these pages naturally augments the first two elements of trust and love as the desired results inevitably begin to show up.

These three factors of trust, love, and integrity are wholly integral and interdependent toward the accomplishment of hair recovery. With accomplishment comes the final element, peace.

The transformation of your body, and specifically the hair on your head, requires a feat of courage and faith. This can be more than a little frightening for some people who suffer from hair loss or damage. Until this instant, you may only have experienced discouragement and doubt.

Just consider for one brief minute that the only thing that may be blocking you from recovering your crown of glory is just that: discouragement and doubt. These feelings, which are totally valid, and perhaps quite justified, may in fact be the very things that keep you from achieving your goals. Think back on how often you've heard of a remedy for your particular malady, then tried it and failed, or didn't give it a shot at all. There may just be a seed of doubt taking root on some level in your mind. Take a look and see if it isn't there...

And then consider that true courage comes from the willingness to face your fears and doubts head-on by acknowledging them—and acting anyway. Perhaps Euripides defined it best almost 2,500 years ago when he said that courage is "to bear unflinchingly what heaven sends."

The advice conveyed within these pages has, hopefully, given you enough information to reason with your fears, surmount them, and commit to the program. Results always begin with a commitment. Nothing was ever achieved in human history without this critical step. Ask yourself now, are you willing to set aside your fears, trepidation, skepticism, or past failures and misfires and make a commitment anyway? If the answer is yes, then read the following contract. Type it out, or write it on a piece of parchment or card stock. Feel free to modify it, if you'd like. Sign it and date it, then post it somewhere where you can see it (*i.e.*, your office at home or your bathroom). Whenever you begin to doubt yourself, come back and visit it for a dose of en*courage*ment.

CONTRACT FOR COURAGE AND FAITH

I, _____, understand that I am committing myself to an act of courage and faith by undertaking this 7-Step Program for a minimum of 90 days, and ideally for one year. I commit myself to faithfully fulfilling the requirements of the program from _____ to
_____.   *today's date*
one year from today.

I, _____, further acknowledge and understand that this program requires dedication, perseverance, and the courage to keep going to produce the results I desire. I, _____, pledge to take excellent care of my mind, body, and spirit—plenty of rest, exercise, nutrition, play, and spiritual practice—for the entire term of this program.

*Signature*_____   _____

*Date*_____

As Mark Twain once said, "Courage is resistance to fear, mastery of fear—not *absence* of fear." Congratulations! In spite of your feelings, you have set yourself on the brave road to recovery, on the path to a transformation of your life.

A word of prudence, though: commitment comes and goes as surely as your emotions swell and dip. It is necessary to acknowledge this, too. After all, you are human, so remember also to have compassion for yourself. Embrace your humanity, and be aware of the instances when your commitment wanes. That is when you want to refer back to your contract.

Now that you are committed, there is only one thing left—action, the sister element to commitment in producing results. The best advice here is to simply take it one day at a time. Focus only on the here and now—the present. For that is all that really matters, isn't it? What are you doing in the present moment, on this present day? Putting your attention on all the activities you have scheduled tomorrow, next week, or next month will only tend to overwhelm you. Similarly, placing your thoughts on what you did yesterday or how you didn't do so well last week doesn't serve you either. Nothing will, and nothing *can*, serve you more than simply being mindful of today. After all, isn't the past already here and gone? Isn't the future already on its way? Has it ever needed your assistance in getting here?

Plan ahead to stay with the program, but give yourself the gracious gift of taking it in single, manageable, one-day segments. Gradually, over time, you will see remarkable results. The fears, doubts, skepticism, and cynicism will fade with the recovery of your crown of glory. Ever-increasing excitement, confidence, and gratification will displace those old, familiar feelings. That is perhaps the greatest benefit of this program, one that has been hardly touched upon in these pages. By healing your hair loss or damage, you are also healing your inner self, reconnecting with your potential for joy, living, and self-expression.

Trust. Love. Integrity. Peacc.

Appendix 1:

Riquette's *Cuisine de Beauté*

In my basic 7-Step Program, I have given you recipes that use a very select group of powerful natural ingredients known through the ages for their restorative, healing properties. Believe me, narrowing down my choices and deciding which of the recipes in my arsenal of treatments would be most effective, simplest to prepare, and easiest to use, proved to be a very difficult task. I wanted to share with you every single one of the treatments and products I have in my recipe file!

When I came to my senses, I decided I would give you the basic program that will provide you with results and then supplement it with the following "graduate course" in the use of herbs, with recipes that employ many other wonderful gifts of nature. Even this barely scratches the surface of available compounds!

Do not use these recipes during the first 90 days of your program, with the exception of the natural coloring treatments, that you might want to use to darken your new hair as it begins to grow, making it more visible. These natural coloring rinses are the *only* supplementary treatments that you may use right now. Stick to the original plan without fail, and without any additions and changes. You have a lifetime ahead of you to play with new, natural treatments.

Here I will give you alternative treatments that retard balding and encourage new growth. I have also included some new treatments that you can add to your routine. Before I give you the recipes, I want to share the following list of nature's gifts for your hair and skin. I have broken these herbs, flowers, roots, and other organic botanical treasures down by use—conditioners, dandruff treatments, and treatments for oiliness or dryness, for example.

After you have completed the 7-Step Program, you may mix and match ingredients in the recipes. For example, you might try adding nettles to the infusion used in your Scalp Shampoo, or substitute a decoction of quassia chips for the boiling water that moistens the fuller's earth and henna for the weekly Mud Pack.

Brunettes might want to add cloves, coffee, or raspberry to the infusion used to make the Protective Sealing Lotion; cowslip, marigolds, or yarrow could add life to blond or golden hair.

Natural Hair Care Ingredients

Conditioners:		
Basil oil	Nettle and cherry	Ragwort
Cherry bark	bark infusion	Rosemary
Lavender oil		(leaves and oil)
Dandruff:		
Artichoke	Lemon juice	Orange peel
Bergamot vinegar	Lemon oil	Quassia chips
Chamomile	Mint vinegar	Rosemary
Juniper leaves	Nettle	Soap root
Lemongrass		Willow

Dryness:

Acacia	Comfrey root	Elderflower
Chamomile	Cowslip	Orange flower
Clover		Peach flower

General Care:

Avocado oil	Jaborandi	Parsley
Almond oil	Kelp	Pineapple juice
Beets	Lemongrass	Rosemary
Black currant	Lemon oil	Southernwood
Brewer's yeast	Maidenhair fern	Vinegar (apple cider
Burdock root	Nettle	or white, depending
Dandelion	Olive oil	upon hair color)
Dulse	Onion juice	Walnut oil
Elderflower		Yarrow

To Stimulate Growth:

American bearsfoot	Lady's smock	Onion juice
Basil oil	Lavender oil	Rosemary leaves
Jaborandi	Lemon oil	Southernwood
	Nettle	

To Dislodge Oils Causing Hair Loss:

Basil oil	Nettle	Sage and borax
Governadora	Peach	Southernwood
Lavender oil	Rosemary	
	(leaves and oil)	

Oiliness:

Bergamot	Orrisroot	Rosebuds
Lemongrass	Peppermint oil	White willow bark
Lemon peel	Quassia chips	Witch hazel bark

For Irritated, Sensitive Scalp:

Birch bark	Rosemary	Speedwell
Horsetail	(oil and leaves)	Yarrow

Shine:		
Chamomile	Marigold	Raspberry
Lemon peel	Nettle	Rosemary
Maidenhair fern		Sage

Split Ends:		
Almond oil	Nutmeg oil	Peanut oil
Basil oil	Olive oil	Rosemary oil
Lavender oil		Walnut oil

Natural Hair Colorings

Make decoctions or infusions of these natural products, then use these liquids to rinse color into your hair. You won't see the immediate results associated with chemical coloring processes, but instead will see gradual color that intensifies with continued use.

Blond or Light:		
Chamomile	Lemon juice	Orange peel
Comfrey root	Lemon peel	Orrisroot
Cowslip flowers	Marigold flowers	White vinegar
Elderflower	Mullein (yellow)	White willow bark
Grapefruit peel		Yarrow

Golden Blond:		
Bedstraw	Chamomile	Henna
Beets		Marigold flowers

Brown or Reddish Brown:		
Beets	Cloves	Indigo
Cinnamon	Coffee	Sage
	Henna	

Brunette:

Apple cider vinegar	Henna	Rosemary
Bergamot	Jaborandi	Sage
Cloves	Nettle	Southernwood
Coffee	Quassia chips	Thyme
	Raspberry	

Natural Skin-Care Ingredients

Acne:

Cantaloupe	Lavender	Papaya
Goldenseal	Mango	Sea salt
Honey		White willow bark

Blackheads:

Buttermilk	Honey	Violet
	Pansy	

Complexion:

Almond milk	Coriander	Rosewater
Caraway	Jamaica flowers	Yogurt
	Parsley	

Dry skin:

Aloe vera	Dandelion	Orange blossom
Anise	Fennel	Orange peel
Apple	Honeydew	Orrisroot
Chamomile	Licorice	Pansy
Caraway	Milk	Parsley
Clover	Mint	Peach
Comfrey	Oatmeal	Strawberry
(leaves and roots)	Olive oil	Violet
Cowslip		Yarrow

Emollients:

Almond oil	Flaxseed oil	Mint
Aloe vera	Glycerine	Oatmeal
Apricot oil	Honey	Orange flowers
Cocoa butter	Lanolin	Quince seeds
Comfrey	Lecithin	Slippery elm
Flax	Malva flowers	Wheat germ oil
	Marshmallow root	

Exfoliants:

Catsfoot	Papaya	Pineapple
Lemon juice		Tomato

Normal Skin:

All fruits	All vegetables	Leek
All grains	Avocado	Peach
	Banana	

Oily Skin:

Anise	Dulse	Lemongrass
Apricot	Fennel	Licorice
Caraway	Lavender	Papaya
Cucumber	Lemon (juice, oil,	Rose
Dandelion	and peel)	Witch hazel

Pimples:

Almond meal	Milk	Peppermint
Comfrey	Oatmeal	Yogurt
	Papaya	

Pores:

Almond meal	Elderflower	Pennyroyal
Buttermilk	Honey	Peppermint
Camphor (oil)	Lavender	Sandalwood
Coltsfoot	Oatmeal	Strawberry
Comfrey	Papaya	Vinegar
Egg white	Parsley	White willow bark
	Peach	

Scaling:

Avocado	Papaya	Salt

Sensitive or Irritated Skin:

Aloe vera	Elderflower	Rose
Avocado	Figwort	Sassafras
Birch bark	Fuchsia	Sorrel
Comfrey	Lavender	Tansy
Cranberry	Marigold	Walnut (leaves, bark)
Egg (inner skin, white)		Yarrow

Tone:

Bay	Honey	Salt
Chamomile	Orange blossoms	Sandalwood
Celery		Vetivert

Plants and Herbs

Open your dictionary and you'll probably find that its definition of the word "plant" probably refers to an organism in the vegetable kingdom with cell walls made of cellulose, and which transmutes inorganic substances (*i.e.*, carbon dioxide) in order to grow. Whatever the definition says, it will hardly do justice to the innumerable variety of species covering the globe, nor even the organisms from the vegetable kingdom we'll be utilizing during this program. Several of the chapters refer to various plants and herbs that are widely known for their properties of stimulating hair growth, restoring vitality, and enhancing the body's performance. It will greatly support your understanding of those plants and herbs by taking a moment to go over their basic physiology and some fundamental ways in which to prepare them for use.

A plant is essentially made up of five parts: roots, stems, leaves, flowers, and fruit. Roots can be found underground, and have two main duties: 1) they anchor the plant into the ground, and 2) they absorb water and nutrients from the soil.

Stems are a bit more complicated. Herbaceous perennials have stems that dwell underground, with roots that extend deeper into the soil from the bottom side of the stem. These kinds of stems are known as *rootstocks*. *Stolon stems* grow on the surface and send their roots down into the ground, much like a rootstock. *Corm stems* are short sticks, or bulbs, that live underground, storing food and producing an *aerial stem*, the type that most people probably think of as a stem (gladiola and tulip bulbs are good examples of corm stems). Aerial stems bear leaves, which supply the plant with food.

Green leaves, through the function of photosynthesis, process the energy of sunlight to combine simple substances absorbed from the soil and air and convert them into complex food matter. During photosynthesis, plants use up carbon dioxide and produce oxygen. Chlorophyll, a critical agent in this process, is the pigment that gives a green leaf its color. There are other pigments, but those colors are masked until the leaf dies and the chlorophyll breaks down.

The botanical function of flowers is reproduction. Born on a receptacle on the stem, the typical flower is made up of several parts: the *calyx*, a set of leaves that protect the flower before it opens; the *corolla*, a set of white or colorful leaves commonly called petals; the *stamen*, which is the male organ that provides fertilization in the form of pollen; and the very center of the flower, which is the *pistil*, the female organ that captures the pollen produced by the stamen.

Fruit has a much more extensive definition in botany than it does in the popular vernacular, but in essence it is the ripened ovary of a flower or flower cluster. Botanically speaking, nuts, beans, corn grains, tomatoes, and dandelion seeds are just as much a fruit as figs, oranges, cherries, and lemons. The primary function of fruit is to disperse seeds through nature's boundless ingenuity in preserving and expanding life: wind, birds, humans, or falling and rolling across the ground.

It has been said that nature provides a remedy for every disease. Over the past twenty years, herbs have grown substantially in repute toward proving this aphorism to be true. To obtain herbs, you can take a trip to the wilds, grow them yourself, pull out the yellow pages and find an herb supplier in your neighborhood, or find a supplier on the Internet. The yellow pages are probably the easiest and quickest, especially since most health food stores, drug stores, and supermarkets now carry extensive supplies of herbs. And the Internet offers hundreds of good companies that sell almost anything you could ever want.

Herbs come in diverse forms, ranging from fresh, dried, or powdered, and can be prepared in many ways to utilize the various parts of these plants. The following types of preparations are the most commonly applied in herbal medicines. Not all of these methods will be employed in this program, but as you explore the world of herbs and their myriad properties, it can be useful information.

Infusion: An infusion is the process of making a tea-like liquid by steeping the plant parts (customarily the green parts or flowers) in boiling water, which extracts their active ingredients. The relatively short exposure to heat minimizes the loss of any vital healing properties. In many formulas, the hot water is poured over the herbs, but some call for the plants to be added to the boiling water; the pot should then be removed from the heat or the heat is reduced, depending upon the recipe. You should use either a glass or enamel pot to steep the plants. Many metal pots will chemically interact with the herbs, negating their active ingredients. While allowing the herbs to steep for approximately 10 minutes, the pot should be covered with a tight-fitting lid to minimize evaporation.

Decoction: This process extracts primarily the mineral salts and bitter essences of herbs and plants, rather than the vitamins and healing properties. This is also the best method to be used when working with roots, bark, wood, and seeds. Most decoction formulas require that you boil about a half-ounce of the plant per one cup of pure water in an enameled or glass pot. Boil them for about 10 minutes, then cover and allow to steep for another 10 minutes. Green plant parts can be added to boiling water and boiled for about 4 minutes before removing from the heat. Then cover and let steep for another 3 minutes. Strain, and then store in a clean glass jar or squeeze bottle.

Cold Extract: Preparation of a cold extract takes a lot longer than an infusion, but it is more effective at extracting and preserving the healing properties. Add about twice the measurement of herbs used in an infusion to cold water in an enameled or glass pot (again, metals can interfere with the herbs). Most formulas require that you let the concoction stand for about twelve hours. Then strain and store in a clean glass jar or squeeze bottle.

Powder: Dried plant parts can be ground with a mortar and pestle to make a powder. This powder can be ingested with water, soups, juice, sprinkled on foods, or inserted into gelatin capsules and swallowed. You should do some research to determine the proper dosages for powder forms of any herb.

Tincture: A tincture is made by combining about 1 to 4 ounces of a powdered herb with about 12 ounces of grain alcohol. Pure water should be added to reduce the alcohol to a 50 percent solution (calculated by knowing what percentage of alcohol solution you started with). Pour into a glass jar with a tight lid, and let stand for one to two weeks depending upon the formula, giving the mixture a good shake once or twice a day. Then strain and store in a clean glass jar or squeeze bottle. The alcohol content will preserve the tincture's healing properties for quite a long time.

Essence: Dissolving an ounce of an herb's essential oil in a pint of grain alcohol (vodka or rum) can make an essence, which is an excellent way of preserving the healing properties in the oils.

Ointment: Mixing one part herbs with four parts hot petroleum jelly can make an ointment. Or you can infuse the herbs in boiling water, strain, then add the decoction to olive oil and simmer until the water has evaporated. Add beeswax for a firm consistency. Continue simmering until the mixture has melted, and stir until well blended. A small amount of gum benzoin, or a drop of tincture of benzoin per ounce, will preserve the ointment.

Poultice: A poultice can be used to apply herbal remedies directly to the skin with moist heat, soothing the body or drawing out impurities. Preparation begins by crushing the curative parts of the plants into a pulpy mass, then moistening with hot water, or combining with a hot mixture of flour or cornmeal. (Use caution, making sure not to burn the skin.) The mixture is best applied by spreading the paste on a soft cloth and then wrapping it around the affected area. The cloth can continually be refreshed by periodically adding additional hot water. Upon removing the poultice, gently wash the skin with warm water to cleanse any remaining residues of the poultice.

Cold Compress: Many herbs can be used topically to heal conditions on the skin or ailments just below the epidermis. A healing cold compress can be made by soaking a towel or cloth in a cool infusion or decoction. Wring out the excess liquid, and apply to the affected area for about 15 to 20 minutes. Reapply with a fresh compress and continue until the ailment is relieved.

Fomentation: A fomentation, or hot compress, is made in the same manner as a cold compress, except that the infusion or decoction is as hot as possible. Use caution, making sure not to burn the skin.

Light and oxygen are the two most formidable adversaries to preserving the effectiveness of herbs. They should be stored in clean, airtight jars made with dark glass and kept in a cool, dry place. Dried herbs will inevitably lose their potency, so they should be replaced after a year.

Appendix 2:

Shopping List for the 7-Step Program

All of these ingredients should be readily available at your local health food store, drug store, or supermarket. These ingredients are for the formulas in the 7-Step Program only. If you're going to mix up other formulas from this book, add those ingredients to this list. With these ingredients, you'll be able to make your first batch of:

- Daytime Scalp Stimulator or
  Alternative (nonalcoholic) Daytime Scalp Stimulator (pages 47–48)

- Nighttime Scalp Stimulator (page 48)

- Super Scalp Stimulator (pages 49–50)

- Slougher Cocktail (pages 51–52)

- Mud Pack (page 53)

- Scalp Shampoo (page 57)

- Hair Shampoo (page 58)

- Protective Sealing Lotion (page 60)

- Tea Rinse (page 60)

Ingredients

Rosemary oil (6-10 teaspoons)

Basil oil (3-5 teaspoons)

Lavender oil (3 teaspoons)

Lemon oil (2 teaspoons)

White iodine (1 teaspoon—
more if you're using the
Alternative (nonalcoholic)
Daytime Scalp Stimulator)

Castor oil (½ teaspoon—
more if you're using the
Alternative (nonalcoholic)
Daytime Scalp Stimulator)

Vodka (¼ cup + a fifth)

Aspirin tablets (10)

Alka-Seltzer tablets (2)

Cayenne pepper (1 teaspoon)

Fuller's earth (1 cup)

Neutral henna (1 cup)

Basil leaves
(3 heaping tablespoons crushed)

Lavender flowers
(1 heaping tablespoon)

Rosemary leaves
(3 heaping tablespoons)

Liquid castile soap (1 cup) or
4 tablespoons soapwort

Nettles (3 heaping tablespoons)

Sage (3 heaping tablespoons)

Chamomile flowers
(2 heaping tablespoons)

Dried horsetail (1 tablespoon)

Indian hemp (1 tablespoon)

Chaparral (1 tablespoon)

32 ounces apple cider vinegar

Appendix 3: Daily Log

	Sunday	Monday	Tuesday
Morning	• Before shower, brush body with a loofah for 5 minutes • Massage scalp for 5 minutes • Brush hair for 50 strokes • Shampoo with Scalp Shampoo and Hair Shampoo • Morning Scalp Stimulator *Juice* *Breakfast/protein shake*	• 20 minutes of exercise • 20 minutes of meditation • Before shower, brush body with a loofah for 5 minutes • Massage scalp for 5 minutes • Brush hair for 50 strokes • Shampoo with Scalp Shampoo and Hair Shampoo. • Morning Scalp Stimulator *Juice* *Breakfast/protein shake*	• 20 minutes of exercise • 20 minutes of meditation • Before shower, brush body with a loofah for 5 minutes • Massage scalp for 5 minutes • Brush hair for 50 strokes • Shampoo with Scalp Shampoo and Hair Shampoo • Morning Scalp Stimulator *Juice* *Breakfast/protein shake*
Mid-morning	• 20 minutes of exercise. • Massage shoulders and neck to relieve tension • 20 minutes of meditation Snack: *half of a protein bar* *1 cup nonfat yogurt*	• Massage shoulders and neck to relieve tension Snack: *half of a protein bar* *1 cup nonfat yogurt*	• Massage shoulders and neck to relieve tension. Snack: *fruit*
Noon hour	Eat lunch • Massage scalp for 5 minutes	Eat lunch • Massage scalp for 5 minutes	Eat lunch • Massage scalp for 5 minutes
Mid-afternoon	Snack	Snack	Snack
Evening	Eat dinner • Massage scalp for 5 minutes • Brush hair for 50 strokes • Wash hairbrush. • Slougher Cocktail • Mud Pack • Protein Pack	Eat dinner • Massage scalp for 5 minutes • Brush hair for 50 strokes • Nighttime Scalp Stimulator • Wash hairbrush	Eat dinner • Massage scalp for 5 minutes • Brush hair for 50 strokes • Nighttime Scalp Stimulator • Wash hairbrush

Wednesday	Thursday	Friday	Saturday
• 20 minutes of exercise • 20 minutes of meditation • Before shower, brush body with a loofah for 5 minutes • Massage scalp for 5 minutes • Brush hair for 50 strokes • Shampoo with Scalp Shampoo and Hair Shampoo • Morning Scalp Stimulator	• 20 minutes of exercise • 20 minutes of meditation. • Before shower, brush body with a loofah for 5 minutes • Massage scalp for 5 minutes • Brush hair for 50 strokes • Shampoo with Scalp Shampoo and Hair Shampoo • Morning Scalp Stimulator	• 20 minutes of exercise • 20 minutes of meditation • Before shower, brush body with a loofah for 5 minutes • Massage scalp for 5 minutes • Brush hair for 50 strokes • Shampoo with Scalp Shampoo and Hair Shampoo • Morning Scalp Stimulator	• 20 minutes of exercise • 20 minutes of meditation • Before shower, brush body with a loofah for 5 minutes • Massage scalp for 5 minutes • Brush hair for 50 strokes • Shampoo with Scalp Shampoo and Hair Shampoo • Morning Scalp Stimulator
Juice *Breakfast/protein shake*	*Juice* *Breakfast/protein shake*	*Juice* *Breakfast/protein shake*	*Juice* *Breakfast/protein shake*
• Massage shoulders and neck to relieve tension	• Massage shoulders and neck to relieve tension	• Massage shoulders and neck to relieve tension	• Massage shoulders and neck to relieve tension
Snack: *half of a protein bar* *1 cup nonfat yogurt*	Snack: *half of a protein bar* *1 cup nonfat yogurt*	Snack: *half of a protein bar* *1 cup nonfat yogurt*	Snack: *half of a protein bar* *1 cup nonfat yogurt*
Eat lunch • Massage scalp for 5 minutes	Eat lunch • Massage scalp for 5 minutes	Eat lunch • Massage scalp for 5 minutes	Eat lunch • Massage scalp for 5 minutes
Snack	Snack	Snack	Snack
Eat dinner • Massage scalp for 5 minutes • Brush hair for 50 strokes • Nighttime Scalp Stimulator • Super Scalp Stimulator • Wash hairbrush	Eat dinner • Massage scalp for 5 minutes • Brush hair for 50 strokes • Nighttime Scalp Stimulator • Wash hairbrush	Eat dinner • Massage scalp for 5 minutes. • Brush hair for 50 strokes • Nighttime Scalp Stimulator • Wash hairbrush	Eat dinner • Massage scalp for 5 minutes • Brush hair for 50 strokes • Nighttime Scalp Stimulator • Wash hairbrush

Tips:

- Take a picture of your hair every month. Be proud of your progress.
- Create an affirmation for yourself and say it after your meditation. Change your affirmation every month.
- Exercise every day for 20 minutes.
- Meditate every day for 20 minutes.
- Get a Magic Haircut every month.
- Do not wear a wig, hairpiece, cap, or hat.
- Do not pull hair tight or part it.
- Do not brush hair when it is wet.
- Make mittens out of old towels to dry hair.
- Pull hair gently to bring blood flow to roots of hair.
- Finish off with a cool rinse after shampooing.
- Color hair naturally and avoid any chemical treatments.
- Create a poster with different hairstyles.
- Drink at least 8 glasses of water a day.
- Change your pillowcases every week.

Appendix 4: Before and After Photos

Before

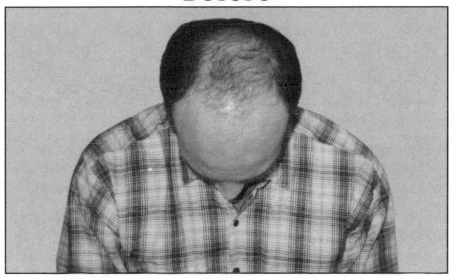

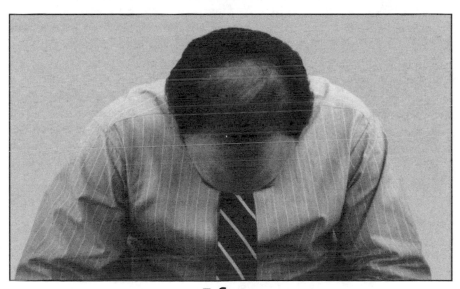

After

Before

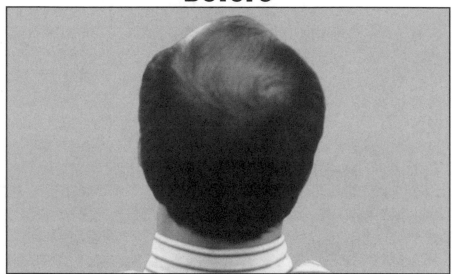

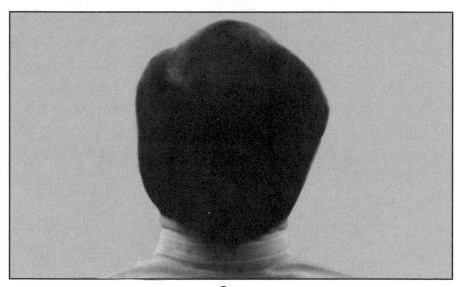

After

Before

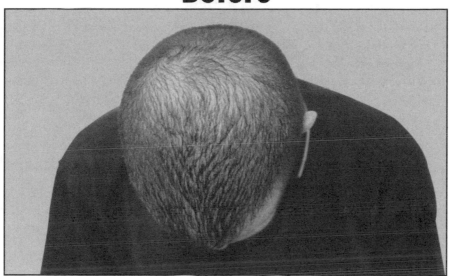

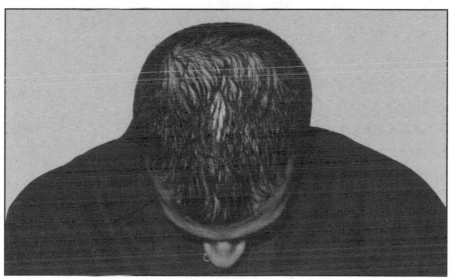

After

Before

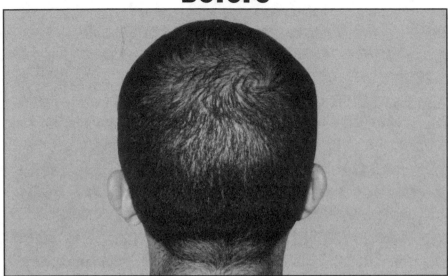

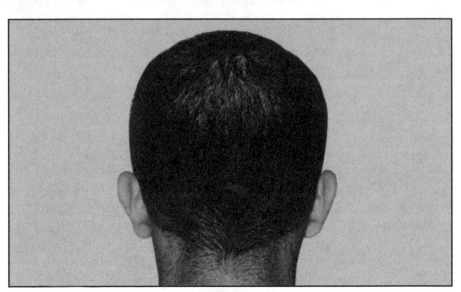

After

Before

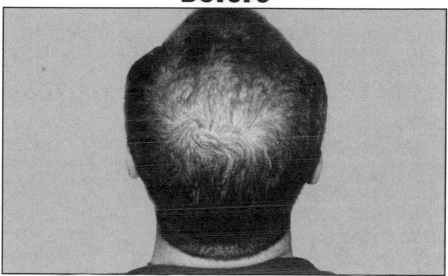

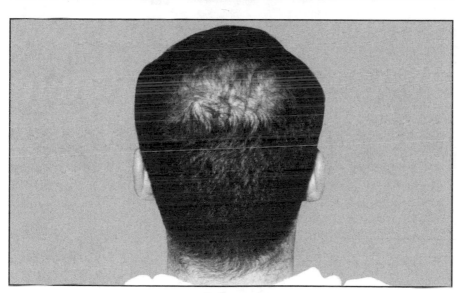

After

Before

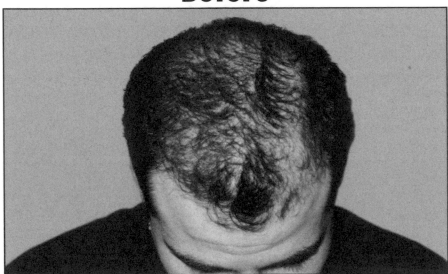

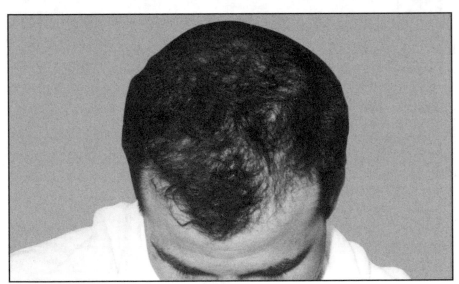

After

Index

About the Author

S ince opening that little shop in Rose Bay Sydney back in 1969, Riquette's business has blossomed beyond her wildest dreams. Her reputation for helping people has grown to world-renowned status. She has appeared on countless radio shows, and been published in hundreds of newspapers and magazines (*Harper's Bazaar*, *Vogue*, *Entrepreneur*, *Allure*, *Weight Watchers*, *People*, *The National Examiner*, and even *Beverly Hills, 90210— The Official Magazine,* to name a few). She has appeared repeatedly on such television shows as *The Tonight Show with Johnny Carson* and *Late Night with David Letterman* and has been a guest on *CNN*, *Live with Regis and Kathie Lee*, *Sally Jessy Raphael*, *The Maury Povich Show*, *Body By Jake*, *CBS This Morning*, *Hour Magazine*, and even had some fun with Don Rickles on *The Merv Griffin Show*. She travels throughout North America, Europe, the Far East, and Australia, speaking and making media appearances. She lectures for corporations and organizations such as United Airlines, General Motors, Christian Dior, the American Cancer Society, Saks Fifth Avenue, governmental agencies, and hospitals. *Grow Hair Fast* is Riquette's third book on hair loss. She is also the author of *Kitchen Cosmetics* and *International Beauty Secrets*. Riquette currently lives and works in Los Angeles.